THE DIGESTIVE CONTRACT

Intestinal Microbiology and Probiotics

Professor (D[r] med) M F Kirkman

With contributions from

Dr Lennart Cedgard M.D.
(Clinical Probiotic Protocols)

Bio Pathica Ltd

Professor (D^r med) Michael Kirkman

1st Edition 2002

Published by Bio Pathica Ltd,
PO Box 217, Ashford, Kent, TN23 6ZU, England

ISBN 0-9543405-0-7

The Authors wish to acknowledge the work of Faye Ballard in the production of this volume; and of Duncan Greenaway B.A. (Hons) Architecture who initialised the diagram concepts prior to their production for the book, and to Roger Wilson, Managing Director, Bio Pathica Ltd, for his constant support throughout the research and writing periods of this book.

MFK/LC

Contents

Foreword

My labrador recently developed diarrhoea. At the visit to the vet I relayed the history and outlined his diet. Without hesitation the vet concluded: 'He's got a dysbiosis, causing leaky gut and has developed a wheat sensitivity. Take him off wheat for a while and give him this probiotic"

Dysbiosis? Leaky Gut? Probiotic? To most *medical* practitioners these concepts are unknown, or if they have heard of these terms they won't know what they mean nor the importance of them in the causation of chronic disease.

As this is being written a research project is starting at Manchester's Wythenshaw hospital into a 'new' treatment for childhood eczema which is being hailed as a 'cure'. What is the wonder drug? - a probiotic. One of a group of natural medicines sold in health food stores for decades, but ignored by the medical establishment. The study follows research in Finland which showed that giving probiotics to a mother prior to birth and then to the baby halved the incidence of eczema.

Eighteen years of practice in complementary medicine has increasingly shown me the importance of the digestive system and diet in health, and this applies not only to disorders of digestion, but also of apparently unrelated conditions. Eczema, arthritis, migraine and chronic fatigue commonly have digestive problems as the underlying cause - and if this is adequately treated results in resolution of the problem.

Most patients with disturbance of bowel function, abdominal discomfort and excess flatulence are commonly diagnosed with 'irritable bowel' and given symptomatic treatment such as antispasmodics, only. To my mind irritable bowel is a 'dustbin diagnosis' in that it fobs off the patient with no diagnosis at all, just a description of symptoms. All patients with irritable bowel have a dysbiosis, with many subsequently developing leaky gut syndrome and/or candidiasis. These are the true diagnoses, and with correct treatment are curable rather then just treatable by reducing symptoms.

One of the commonest causes of dysbiosis is unnecessary or excessive antibiotic treatment. Antibiotics are prescribed often when there is no evidence of bacterial infection and no investigation to support their use. The result is that the balance of normal, *essential* bacteria in the intestine is affected and a dysbiosis develops, laying the foundation for the development further of a leaky gut or a yeast overgrowth. It is impossible to assess to what extent such 'treatment' has, in fact, *caused* chronic conditions, but it must run into millions. The cost of this hidden epidemic has to be vast, not only in financial terms but in the inferior *quality* of life for the sufferers.

As the Greek physicians recognised we are what we eat (or, more accurately, we are what we *absorb*). The conditions discussed in this book invariably lead to altered absorption, so clearly can affect health in ways unrelated to digestion. Mineral and vitamin deficiencies are common sequelae, and leaky gut causes changing and increasing food sensitivities.

So this book could not be more needed. It sets out in language which is readable for both the practitioner and the patient the symptoms, altered physiology, biochemistry and microbiology of these digestive disturbances. Advice is given on self-recognition of a problem and ideas provided on management and treatment. In terms of the potential improvement for the health of the population it has to be a milestone, *if* the contents are accepted and adopted by medical practitioners.

Over the last twenty years acupuncture has gone from being a totally alternative treatment to one which is now accepted and even practised by the medical profession. Other complementary treatments and concepts are making inroads into the medical world. Ideas expressed in this book, although unorthodox at present, could lay the foundation for better treatment of chronic disease.

The unorthodox treatment of today is the orthodox treatment of tomorrow - and this volume drives forward that concept.

Dr David Dowson

Introduction : Probiotic and Prebiotic Parameters Dietetics and Adjuvants

"Man cannot be completely seen separate from mankind, nor mankind separate from all life, nor life separate from the Universe."

Teillard de Chardin

"Our mode of life itself, the way we live, is emerging as today's principal cause of illness" -

this poignant statement of D[r] Joel Elkes Professor of Behavioural Medicine USA succinctly sets the scene for the Introduction on Probiotic and Prebiotic parameters, dietetics and adjuvants.

Firstly, in order to enhance understanding, some definitions relevant to the text of this book:

a) Nutrients are any substances (including water and functional foods - see later) ingested, absorbed, assimilated, and utilised by an organism in the processes of maintaining growth, repair, healthy structure and function, immune system integrity and vital activities.

b) Nutrition is the science of food, the materials or nutrients in food, what they do, how they interact, all in relation to health. Bio-individuality factors such as age, metabolism, activity and lifestyle levels must be taken into account in nutritional assessment and nutritional 'engineering'.

c) Diet is the general selection of various available foods which are eaten by a person, an area, or ethnic population in a normal process of feeding or living. A balanced diet is a diet of daily/weekly food intake, designed to provide ALL the nutrients in sufficient quantity, quality and absorbability to maintain optimum bodily structure and integrity of function. Such a diet must provide all the necessary nutrients to ensure the body's ability to manufacture the biological molecules for the micro-systems of immune system competence.

Dietetics is the science of ensuring a person eats a balanced diet according to need and bio-individuality status, resulting in total health of body structure and function. Today, the emphasis is towards healthy eating a diet which is rich in whole 'natural' or 'raw' and unprocessed foods; this leads to maximum intestinal function and hence, as will be emphasised in this volume, total Immune System Function. Unfortunately, the polluted world has devastating effects and powerful negative influences in the sphere of nutritional and intestinal health, as are also the effects of leaching of soils and techno-agriculture practices of mass production and use of artificial fertilisers, herbicides and pesticides. These all negate total nutrition as nutrients become depleted in food and toxins are taken in.

A poem (prophetic) of Lord Dunsany (1878 - 1957),

> "When man has poisoned all the flowers,
> And stilled the insects glee,
> And killed the birds with spray that showers
> Our fields with chemistry,
> In his well regulated bowers,
> How lonely man will be"

(written over 50 years ago) comes to mind.

d) Functional Foods - (also known as nutraceuticals) are foods which possess 'bio-activity' and contain (in adequate concentration) one or a combination of nutrient components which affect function in the body, so as to have positive cellular or physiological effects (Roberfroid 1996).

Recent knowledge in bio-science supports the hypothesis that diet also controls and modulates various functions in the body, so as to contribute to the maintenance of a state of good health and reduce the risk of some diseases.

'Research and development of 'functional food' is part of the science of nutrition and the benefit associated with its intake has to be evaluated in the context of diet. The strategy for research and development of a 'functional food' requires:

1) the demonstration of an interaction of a function or functions in the body

2) some understanding of the mechanism thereof

3) the establishment of the effect in relevant biological systems

4) the formulation of sound hypotheses

5) the testing of these hypotheses in human nutrition studies"
(Roberfroid)

The prebiotics, probiotics, symbiotics and adjuvants discussed in this book, fulfil the above criteria.

e) Prebiotic - 'a non -digestible food ingredient that beneficially affects the host by selectively stimulating the growth and/or activity of one or a limited number of bacteria in the colon (Gibson & Roberfroid 1995).

Examples are the non-digestible oligosaccharides (FOS) (inulin and its enzymic hydrolysate oligofructose) and chicory fructose. Prebiotics occur naturally in wheat, Jerusalem artichoke, banana, onion, leek, garlic and chicory.

Although FOS are not digestible in the upper gastrointestinal tract (GI), they do have calorific value. FOS are metabolised by certain intestinal microflora and they also enhance the growth of these beneficial micro-organisms in the intestinal environment (especially the bifido bacteria and lactobacillus - see later). This metabolism process results in energy for the host together with organic acids which become available for absorption and further metabolisation.

Interestingly, there are certain beneficial physiological effects which have been associated directly with FOS consumption and fermentation by intestinal bacteria:-

a) Selective stimulation of growth of bifido bacteria, and hence enhanced populations, also of lactobacilli and similar acid producing bacteria; producing lactic acid and short-chain carboxylic acids (SCFAs).

b) FOS behave like soluble fibre, producing a matrix for the bacteria while also increasing bowel motility and reducing high levels of cholesterol, total LDL, including serum triglycerides and phospho-lipids.

c) Reduction of the risk of developing pre-cancerous lesions in the colon. The incidence of aberrant crypt foci induced by colon carcinogens such as azoxymethane, dimethylhydrazine and perhaps nitrites and nitrates is reduced. Furthermore, inulin stimulates sulphomucin production, and regresses sialo-mucin, such effects are known to reduce colon cancer risk.

d) Improvement of calcium bio-availability, as also magnesium, and the iron and zinc balance without having significant effect on copper bio-availability (Delzemme et al 1995).

e) Observed beneficial effects resulting from increased levels of Bifido-bacteria and Lactobacilli, which occupy more of the 'micro-ecological niches'. Bacteria considered to be undesirable such as E.coli, Salmonella and Clostridium perfringens tend to be excluded. Equally, the production of putrefactive substances, e.g. Phenol, cresol, and indole is decreased, thereby reducing the strain at liver level for detoxification of such substances.

Thus, various potential health benefits of FOS could be a reduction in the risk of intestinal infectious diseases, cardio-vascular diseases, non-insulin dependant diabetes, obesity, osteoporosis and cancer.

An early example of a prebiotic is lactulose, which was used to increase numbers of Bifido-bacteria in bottle-fed infants, though it is also beneficial for intestinal lactic acid bacteria. Related lactose derivatives such as lactitol, a similar disaccharide analogue, have similar effects, and take us into the relatively new science of glycobiology, and various oligosaccharides which contain xylose, mannose, galactose, soya (glyco protein derivatives), and maltose.

Important developments lead toward the use of prebiotics which possess multiple biological functions, including blocking potential adhesion sites of pathogens e.g. Oligosaccharides that have mannose side chains may be effective against Escherichia coli and related organisms.

A Finnish study at University Hospital TURKU produced "clear benefits to the subjects with constipation using a mixture of lactulose and Lactobacillus acidophilus in a fibre enriched yoghurt".

Professor Conn's published works from Yale University School of Medicine puts forward other roles for prebiotics primarily lactulose (galactoside - fructose - synthetic) and raffinose and stachyose - natural in beans:-

a) <u>Lactulose as a cathartic and laxative agent</u> - by stimulating bowel activity and creating acid-induced catharsis. Shown to be a safe cathartic agent in randomised trials for elderly, children, pregnant women and terminally ill. Lactulose, especially in conjunction with lactic acid bacteria, is an effective stool softener, and thus reduces pain on defecation, including cases of acute diverticulitis, as well as before and after haemorrhoidectomy and other types of rectal surgery.

b) Lactulose in the eradication of Salmonella carrier states - especially post-antibiotics and again with lactic acid bacteria. It is important to note that Salmonella bacteria are more comfortable in neutral or alkaline environment and do NOT grow where pH is less than 4.5; but the lactulose, lactic acid and short chain fatty acids (SCFAs) seem to produce an acidity sufficient to kill them off, while avoiding the possibility of resistant strains from long-term antibiotic usage. A similar picture emerges from lactulose/lactic acid bacteria in the Shigella species (dysentery) states.

c) Lactulose and lactic acid bacteria in the prevention of bacterial infections in care home/long stay hospitalised, especially geriatric patients - 2 placebo controlled studies confirm this situation; and both bacteraemic and urinary infections were reduced.

d) Lactulose in prevention of the formation of gallstones especially cholesterol gallstones. Again the synergism of lactic acid bacteria and lactulose produce intestinal acidosis which inhibits the growth of anaerobic enteric bacteria and thus opposes gallstone formation. Also, the prebiotic and enhanced dietary fibre levels, together with the L.A. Bacteria have been shown to reduce bile cholesterol levels.

e) Prevention of colon carcinoma by lactulose. Secondary bile acids such as des-oxycholate acid (DCA) and lithocholic acid have been implicated in colonic carcinogenesis - however lactulose can reduce such formation, probably by reducing the luminal pH; while also a trial indicated that lactulose reduced the recurrence rate of colorectal polyps, especially if accompanied by the concurrent administration of antioxidant vitamins A and E (Roncucci 1993).

f) Lactulose - endotoxin antagonist - especially galactosamine implicated in hepatotoxicity as are other endotoxins (see later).

In the Heel, Ordinatio Anti Homotoxica et Materia Medica, based on the studies of Dr H. H. Reckeweg, it is advocated that Microbiological Therapy has a parallel role within his System of Medicine of Homotoxicology and Anti-Homotoxic Therapy, formulated in 1952 - in principle thus:

"According to Homotoxicology all of those processes, syndromes and manifestations, which we designate as diseases, are the expression thereof that the body is combating poisons (external and internal toxins) and that it wants to neutralise and excrete those poisons. The body either wins or loses the fight thereby. Those processes are always biological, i.e. natural teleological processes, which serve (provide) poison defence and detoxification."

g) Symbiosis - this term was defined in 1879 by Anton Heinrich de Bary as the "continual close-knit cohabitation of organisms of diverse designation". This definition of symbiosis encompasses a great number of life-partnerships including parasitism, neutralism, commensalism and mutualism. In 1951, in this respect, "the value of this interpretation lies in the expansion of the concept of the structural entity of an organism to include heterogenic systems which operate conjointly as a functional unit or field".

Applying this concept to populations of microflora within the alimentary tract - the human/microbial intestinal microflora correlation corresponds perfectly with the definition of a symbiotic partnership. Human microflora, if well established, also contains opportunistic pathological agents with which the body maintains a status of continuous, close cohabitation. These agents are normally kept in check by neutral, commensal and mutualistic micro-organisms and are thus uncapable of developing their disease promoting properties.

h) Symbiotics (Dr Lennart Cedgard - Wasa Medicals) are products in which both a prebiotic and a probiotic are combined in a single product. Symbiotics are defined as 'a mixture of a probiotic and a prebiotic that beneficially affects the host by improving the survival and the implantation of live microbial dietary supplements in the GI tract, by selectively stimulating the growth, and/or by activating the metabolism of one of a limited number of health promoting bacteria' (Roberfroid University of Louvain, Belgium). Such possess positive physiological effects, which may in turn reduce the risk of cancer and heart disease.

i) Probiotics

1/ 'A probiotic agent is a microbial preparation containing live and/or killed microbes, including any constituent parts or metabolic products thereof. Probiotic agents may be employed as food additives, preventative substances or therapeutic agents'.

Institute for Micro-ecology, Old Herborn University 1994

2/ 'A live microbial feed supplement which beneficially affects the host animal (and human) by improving its microbial balance.'

Fuller 1992

3/ 'Naturally existing, or indigenous 'friendly' live bacterial organisms, which contribute to the health and balance of human and animal GI tracts by providing protection against toxins and disease, and by improving intestinal function, nutritional and immune system status.'

Kirkman 1999

The majority of probiotics contain Lactobacillus species and Bifido bacterium species; but Dr Goldum of Tufts University School of Medicine lists Streptococcus species including Streptococcus Thermophilus, Enterococcus species and others that have been successfully utilised as functional probiotics.

Lactobacillus GG (LGG) has been extensively researched and hailed since its discovery from a human faecal culture by Gorbach and Goldin (GG) in 1985 and is now a widely used probiotic - it is a L. Rhamnosum species.

A recent meeting in Bonn, Germany October 1998, the proceedings of which were published in 'Immunology Today September 1999 (Vol. 20, No 9, 387)", focused attention on the Imm uno-regulatory properties of probiotics with the aim of identifying their cellular and molecular mechanisms of action. This MUST now be included in the definition.

This symposium concluded with 12 suggested health effects of Probiotics:

1/ Increased nutritional value (better digestibility, increased absorption of minerals and vitamins)
2/ Promotion of intestinal lactose digestion
3/ Positive influence of intestinal flora (especially post-antibiotics or radiation induced colitis)
4/ Prevention of intestinal tract infections (bacteria or virus induced, Candida enteritis, Helicobacter pyloris ulcer/neoplasia)
5/ Regulation of gut motility (constipation, irritable bowel syndrome)
6/ Immune System enhancement
7/ Prevention of cancer
8/ Reduction of catabolic products eliminated by kidney and liver
9/ Prevention of Atherosclerosis (reduction of serum cholesterol)
10/ Prevention of osteoporosis
11/ Better development (growth)
12/ Improved well being

Probiotics, in addition, have been given claims of being valid for diarrhoea's (antibiotic induced, travellers and infantile); and for vaginitis (local application) and alcohol-induced liver disease.

Apart from stabilising the flora, probiotics serve to help indigenous flora to recolonise after antibiotic usage, for treatment of food allergies and leaky-gut syndrome (see later). An interesting prospect (also see later for specific details), probiotics seem to provide for Immuno-modulation (positive) and act as adjuvants for vaccines. This latter has been tested (Isolaune et al 1995) where LGG provided an adjuvant therapy to rotavirus care in children. This is NOT way out, for Ayurvedic physicians have used Dahi or curd for this purpose for 4000 years. Scientifically, it appears that LGG stimulates rotavirus specific IgM secreting cells, while also increasing IgA, and IgM seroconversion and hence producing antibodies to rotavirus and possibly similar food/water pathogenic viruses in baby and infantile diarrhoea's.

In respect of food allergies, especially in infants, it is possible there is a role for LGG in reducing intestinal inflammation from milk protein casein allergic reactions in milk fed infants, while also reducing hypersensitivity reactions and food allergies and resultant atopic eczema. At the same time it appears that lactose intolerance, which causes severe intestinal distress due to bloating, flatulence and abdominal pain resulting from individual low level ß galactsidase (lactase) in young and elderly may be alleviated. Not only do probiotics fulfil this role, but natural yoghurts and curds appear to act similarly in enhanced lactase activity. Also, this situation acts as a marker for the extent of bacterial metabolism in the large bowel as indicated by the amount of hydrogen in the breath and hence degree (i.e. lower hydrogen level) of the extent of lactose metabolised PRIOR TO entering the large intestine. Also, according to Gorbach et al 1987, LGG is effective against relapsing diarrhoea caused by Clostridium difficile produced toxin - a well known food poisoning condition.

I am grateful to Dr Roy Fuller for extracts from his article in Positive Health, 30-09-98, Issue 32, p22-24 for thus:

'How do we know that the gut microflora is doing its job of protecting the host against disease?"

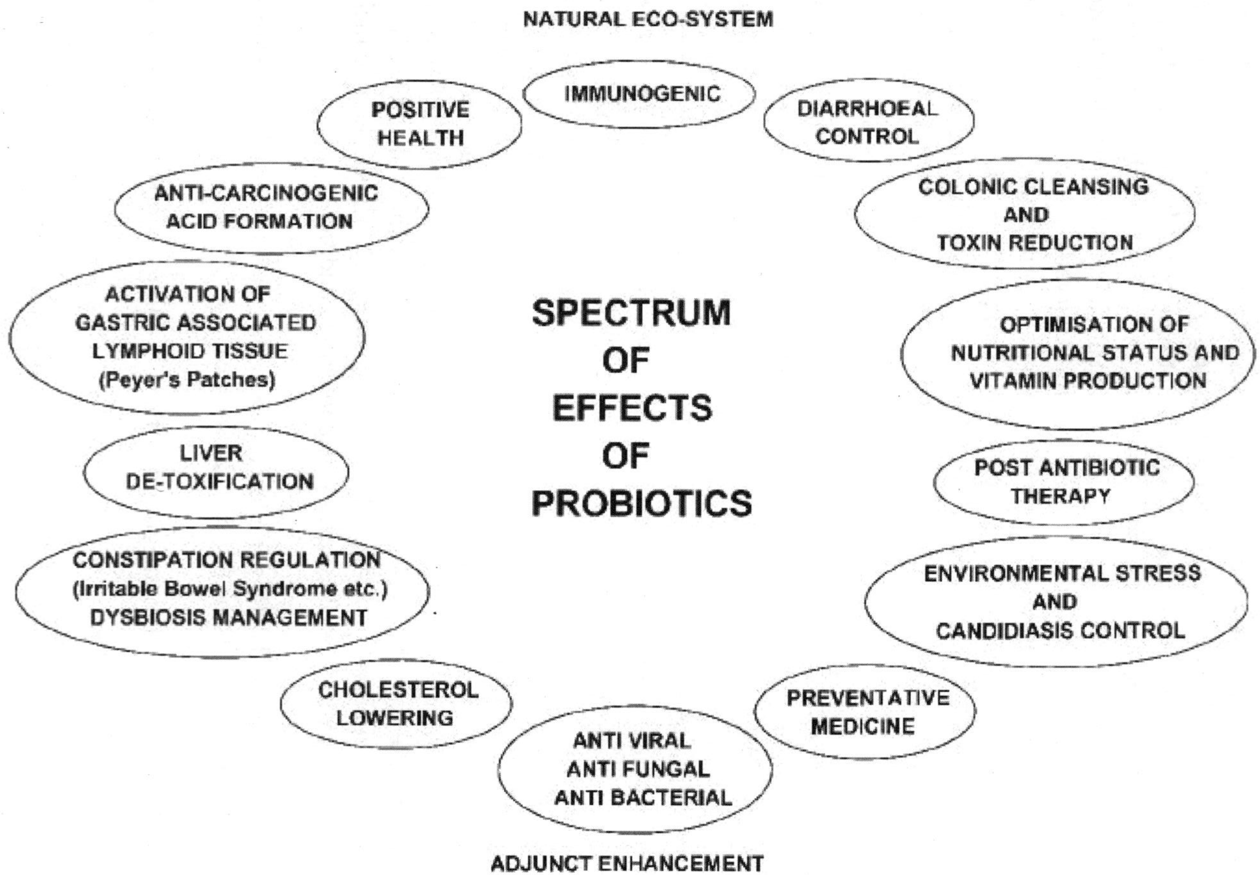
NATURAL ECO-SYSTEM
SPECTRUM OF EFFECTS OF PROBIOTICS
IMMUNOGENIC
DIARRHOEAL CONTROL
COLONIC CLEANSING AND TOXIN REDUCTION
OPTIMISATION OF NUTRITIONAL STATUS AND VITAMIN PRODUCTION
POST ANTIBIOTIC THERAPY
ENVIRONMENTAL STRESS AND CANDIDIASIS CONTROL
PREVENTATIVE MEDICINE
ANTI VIRAL
ANTI FUNGAL
ANTI BACTERIAL
CHOLESTEROL LOWERING
CONSTIPATION REGULATION
(Irritable Bowel Syndrome etc.)
DYSBIOSIS MANAGEMENT
LIVER DE-TOXIFICATION
ACTIVATION OF GASTRIC ASSOCIATED LYMPHOID TISSUE
(Peyer's Patches)
ANTI-CARCINOGENIC ACID FORMATION
POSITIVE HEALTH
ADJUNCT ENHANCEMENT

The evidence comes from three sources:

1. If animals are reared in the complete absence of microbes (germ free) they are more susceptible to diseases such as cholera, dysentery and salmonellosis.

2. Antibiotics given orally often induce diarrhoea. The antibiotic is killing off the protective microbes and allowing dangerous pathogens to multiply.

3. The diarrhoeal conditions induced by antibiotic feeding can be treated, by dosing with an enema prepared from a suspension of faeces from a healthy adult.

The evidence for the protective effect of the gut flora is, therefore, a incontrovertible fact. The aim of probiotics supplements is to ensure that the microbes responsible for the protection are present in the intestine.

How do they work?

Little is known about the way in which probiotics are able to inhibit other micro-organisms in the gut. But we can speculate about how they may be operating by reference to existing knowledge on microbial interaction in the gut.

Probiotics may be having their effect by one or more of the following methods:

1. <u>Competition for nutrients.</u> The gut is such a rich source of nutrients that this seems unlikely, but it should be remembered that it only requires the absence of one essential nutrient to prevent the growth of a micro-organism. There is some evidence that this type of mechanism is at least partly responsible for the inhibition of Cl. difficile by the gut microflora.

2. <u>Direct chemical inhibition.</u> Lactic acid bacteria are known to produce a variety of different antibiotic-like substances. However, their activity in the gut has never been demonstrated and this seems an unlikely explanation.

3. <u>Competition for adhesion sites on the gut wall.</u> Many gut pathogens, in order to colonise the gut, have to attach to the lining of the intestinal

tract. This enables them to survive the flushing effect of peristalsis. If the probiotic organism attaches preferentially to the gut wall and prevents the pathogen adhering, it will be unable to colonise and produce disease. There is good evidence that lactobacilli, commonly used in probiotic preparations, can adhere to the gut wall.

4. Stimulation of immunity. A great deal of work has been done recently in laboratory animals which demonstrates that administration of lactic acid bacteria by mouth can stimulate the immune system. Perdigon and her colleagues in Argentina have shown that the increase in antibody level is related to the reduction in salmonella. Recent work by Nestlé in Switzerland has shown that similar immune responses can be induced in human subjects by administration of L. Acidophilus LC1. The recognition that lactic acid bacteria can stimulate an immune response is a very important finding because it means that there are now mechanisms for the probiotic to have an effect in sites outside the intestinal tract.

The composition of probiotic preparations varies greatly and it is likely that no one mechanism would explain the activity of all probiotics. However, there seems little doubt that one or more of the above suggested mechanisms will be responsible for the antimicrobial activity of many probiotic preparations.

The Heel Ordinatio Anti Homotoxica indicates that die Rote Liste contains approximately 35 microbial preparations, though the majority are 4, i.e. Enterococcus faecalis, Escherichia coli, Bifidobacterium bifidum, Lactobacillus Acidophilus N.B. here, as yet there is no internationally agreed bio-naming standard. Also, and MOST importantly there is the non-symbiotic Saccharomyces boulardii - used successfully in diarrhoea management.

Various sources, especially Kolb, Hans and Maaß (1991) Kompendium de Mikrobiologischen Therapie, indicates that micro-biological therapy has attained scientific substantiation through recent immunological research, such that microbiological therapy seems to work via the liberation of cytokinetic substances, such as interleukin - 1L-1, IL-6 and interferon B which is so stimulated in direct correlation with dosage. Micro-biological preparations activate dormant beta cells (see Mucosal immunity and GALT later) causing these beta cells to proliferate, thereby causing a Cascade Reaction which thereby enhances IgA - synthesis. This stimulation of the activity level in the mucosa immune system is verified by a detectable increase of secretory IgA in the saliva. Thus also, are favourable effects or the psycho-neuro-endocrine-immune system linkages.

Controlled clinical tests have confirmed the indications for microbiological therapy in the following conditions and syndromes:

a) Respiratory - Immuno-modulation

b) Alimentary - Immuno-modulation

1) Gastro-enteritis
2) Entero-colitis
3) Post-antibiotic colitis
4) Ulcerative colitis
5) Crohn's disease
6) Cholecystopathy
7) Mycosis, especially Candida species
8) Leaky-gut syndrome
9) M.E. When due to intestinal origin i.e. Coxsackiae virus, Cytomegalus group of viruses and Epstein-Barr virus and possibly Giardia species. (Anti-homotoxic nosode therapy may be indicated here, but such is outside the scope of this volume)

However, total dietary and nutritional regime is indicated as adjunct therapy, as also is anti-homotoxic detoxification regime (see later) and adequate fluid intake (minimum of 3 litres of water daily) to promote elimination of toxins and to promote renal function.

The preparations Mucosa compositum (for details see The Ordinatio) and Podophyllum compositum are reliable agents in cases displaying colitic symptoms.

Spascupreel (S) is utilised in the treatment of muscle spasm conditions and Vomitusheel (S) is prescribed by general situation of vomiting and nausea (unwellness, feeling sick). There are also many single constituent and combination homoeopathic preparations available e.g. Duodenoheel, Gastricumheel, Hepeel (to aid liver detoxification).

Furthermore, it is MOST important to ensure adequate total nutrient intake in order to allow the body to have available or manufacture all the biological molecular components for optimum immune system competence. Chlorella, Spirulina and Aloe Vera are examples of total nutrient functional foods. It is also important to ensure adequate and various dietary fibre (see later) and sufficient mucus and other types of glycobiologicals.

Finally, in terms of definitions and parameters in this introduction to Intestinal Microbiology and Probiotics, it is time to consider briefly what are perhaps the original natural probiotics - the HSOs or Homeostatic Soil Organisms. I am grateful to Herb Rubin D.C. for some indications on HSOs.

For many years now, the author has been promulgating his Universal Immune Compromisation Syndrome (UICS) hypothesis whereby diseases of plants, animals and humans have become more prevalent (especially infectious viral and bacterial conditions, allergies and post-viral states) in spite of progression in allopathic medicine and surgery, and attention to diet and nutritional supplementation. The author has attributed such to:

a) <u>Exogenous</u> phenomena and toxins
   1) <u>Physical</u> - radiation, microwave, electric and sound (infrasound vibration, low frequency noise, loud noise)
   2) <u>Chemical</u> - pesticides, herbicides, fertilisers, pollutants, food additives and preservatives
   3) <u>Biological</u> - reduction in nutrient and enzyme values of foodstuffs, and increase in processed foods and loss of vitality and SOEFs (Subtle organising energy fields) in organic, natural, raw foods, combined with antibiotics, hormones, vaccines, endocrine disrupters, contaminants in food/water.

b) <u>Endogenous</u> - internal metabolite substances (toxins) and oxidative, lipid peroxidation factors and production of other reactive species.

The author is pleased to note Herb Rubin's thesis along similar lines, leading to understanding of the recent rise in degenerative, chronic and autoimmune conditions, even in children; with each generation becoming weaker than the last. Obviously, individual lifestyles themselves are implicated, as is lack of exercise and the frantic pace of life in the technological age, with domestic, work related and techno-stress predominating. Often such enter the body via antibiotics, cortisone, NSAID's and other drug related nutrient reactions, hormone therapies, excess white sugar, alcohol, carbonated beverages, chlorination and fluorinated water, all act to alter the acid/alkaline balance and hence the indigenous intestinal microflora balance. Thus, the 'friendly' bacteria cannot survive and the environment shifts to favour the 'bad' bacteria, which stress and depress our Immune System competence.

Thus a state of Intestinal Toxaemia becomes the norm and "degeneration begins in the colon" with the following states/syndromes ensuing: chronic fatigue immune deficiency syndromes (CFIDs), hypersensitivity, allergic and asthmatic phenomena, hormonal problems/excesses and deficiencies, especially thymic gland and excessive cortisol (stress hormone) production, the fibromyalgia, arthritides, sciatica and low back pain conditions, diabetes (non-insulin dependent), obesity and high blood pressure states, breast pathology and intestinal states previously outlined. The author has previously attributed most of such to intestinal flora imbalance. Herb Rubin in his purporting of the critical role of HSOs has added in the author's opinion a new valid dimension to the overall disease profile picture.

HSOs play a critical role in universal immune systems structure and function, and help in maintaining bodily homeostasis. Critical today, in so far, as for thousands of years, say 4 million, humans ate fruits and vegetables from soil rich in HSOs which established themselves in the intestine. The HSOs also protected the soil against disease and actually became part of the plants themselves. Today, even in organically grown food, few HSOs exist.

Technically HSOs are natural probiotics which lower the colonic pH and hence favour acid-loving 'friendly' lactobacillus, acidophilus etc., which in turn clear pathogens and yeast's out of the system directly and indirectly; and hence promote nutrient absorption. Originally such natural probiotics were ingested daily in food and were resistant to stomach acid.

HSOs seem to have some unique properties, akin, but variant from modern day probiotics:

1) <u>Stimulation of the body's natural alpha interferon production</u> - which results in regulation of the immune system and anti-viral agents.

2) <u>Stimulation of 'T' and 'B' cells</u> - resulting in 'killing off' of invading agents such as moulds, yeast's, fungi and bacteria while stimulating the B cells to provide a plethora of non-specific, uncoded antibodies.

3) <u>Production of Lactoferrum</u> - HSOs seem to enhance lactoferrum action in protecting the body by reducing invading viruses, parasites and yeast's; and making iron more bio-available.

Thus, considering HSOs is an important concept in Probiotic and Immune System studies and practice of Probiotic Therapy.

The next part of this Introduction considers Probiotics in the context of Natural Therapy and Holistic Health and Holistic Medicine in general.

Lindlahrs definition:

Health = "normal and harmonious vibration of the elements and forces composing the human entity on the physical, mental and moral (spiritual) planes of being, in conformity with the CONSTRUCTIVE PRINCIPLE (The Great Law of Life (NATURE)."

Henri Lindlahr (Philosophy of Natural Therapies)

Holistic Health is a state of mental, physical, emotional psycho-social, spiritual, environmental and lifestyle well-being.

The essence of Holistic Health is a way of living in harmony with self and surroundings. The ability to form and maintain good relationships with others and the ability to cope with and adjust to the many stresses of present-day frantic pace of living in a technological age. Furthermore, it is the state of possessing the strength to eliminate unwanted habits, and the ability to attain spiritual contentment and personal happiness.

This harmony can only be totally attained if every cell in the body has a constant supply of all the correct nutrients in the correct proportions.

Natural therapies have been used to treat disease since our earliest beginning; and from these origins naturopathic medicine has grown and developed. Indeed, the importance of natural therapies is gaining ground in therapeutics today as the long and short term side effects of so many drugs (antibiotics, cortisone derivatives, NSAID'S, etc), become more apparent.

"According to legend, the method of preparing yoghurt was revealed to Abraham by an angel, and he owed his fecundity and longevity to this fermented food. Vedic literature, (6000 BC), from India associates longevity to the consumption of dairy products" (fermented and known as 'curd'). So state Drs Rao and Shahani in J. Of Cultured Dairy Products, (1987-Feb 6-10). The author is most grateful to various Dr K M Shahani's references and publications in the preparation of this booklet, including the cassette-tape recording "Therapeutic Uses of Lactobacillus Acidophilus".

Although lacto-bacillic-fermented foods have been used for ages, the pioneering work of Metchnikoff was perhaps the first to establish that micro-organisms are responsible for the beneficial effects associated with these products (all described in the now rare book (Metchnikoff E. (1908) The prolongation of life - G P Purnam and Sons, New York). This postulates that the intestinal flora produces poisons or ptomaine's, (today we would call these toxins), which can be detrimental to the host. Metchkinoff purported that these harmful effects could be overcome by establishing a specific balance between intestinal bacteria and those found in fermented milk products - the birth of the science of Probiotics!

Recently, it has been determined that the lactobacilli used in the fermentation process of products, such as yoghurt, may improve the nutritional quality as well as the nutritional quantity of the cultured products. This is achieved by increasing the B-vitamin and enzyme contents. In addition, during fermentation the lactobacilli also produce natural antibiotics, natural anti-carcinogenic compounds; together with compounds which retard or inactivate toxins (i.e. natural anti-homotoxicals).

In summary, yoghurt and yoghurt-like products are traditional forms of sour milk consumed in Bulgaria, and now many other countries - the fermentation is brought about by "seeding" evaporated milk with a culture of lacto-bacillus (lactic acid bacilli), and yeast, and allowing it to set at 37°C for 6 to 8 hours. A thick curd is formed - called Dahi in India, where it is used (as for centuries), in preventative medicine and in therapeutic situations. It is important to note the exacting conditions of time, temperature, pH, water content, etc. Such must also prevail and can be monitored in the probiotic manufacture as must be the microbial safety factor.

With his gastro-intestinal microflora man creates a relatively stable 'micro-ecological' system. Within this system every part of the intestinal tract has its own microbial growth. The organospecific type of microflora is generally present in all humans provided no particular conditions exist. Variations of these conditions affect the composition of the microflora, it is particularly susceptible to endogenous and exogenous factors (physical, chemical and biological), its own biochemical processes and its composition in turn influences the metabolism and immunity resistance of the human organism.

Despite some reservations, both qualitative and quantitative, statistically comparable and reproducible findings regarding the typical, normal intestinal microflora in healthy humans are possible. These findings provide the preconditions for the definition of an abnormal intestinal microflora. Also, the results obtained in conventional or gnotobiotic animals enable cautious analogies regarding the multifarious influence of the body flora in humans. Eubiosis is the term for a normal typical settlement of an organ, while abnormal growth is designated 'dysbiosis', and the word 'pro - biotic',(Greek 'for life"), refers to 'friendly' bacteria which contribute so much to the health and the balance of the intestinal tract. "The regular inclusion of friendly bacteria in the diet produces beneficial effects, but since different species differ considerably in the benefits they offer, only selected strains with desirable properties should be selected for supplements" Dr Jeremija Lj RASIC PhD. Novi Sad Institute, Yugoslavia.

So, the many beneficial potentials of the friendly bacteria include detoxification, antibiotic, anti-viral, anti-fungal properties together with anti-stress, anti-carcinogen and immune-enhancing, together with liver stimulating activities. Equally, there appear to be feedback loops to and from via gastrointestinal endocrine - immuno-neuro-psychological pathways, and also through various metabolic pathways.

However, prior to looking at the intestinal microflora and probiotic usage in the context of holistic health and naturopathic medicine, it is important to bear in mind the works of Friend and Shahani - "Commercial preparations of cultures shown to be effective in the laboratory may not contain sufficient viable organisms to be of benefit. Specialised media and techniques are required to handle, propagate and concentrate the lactobacilli to ensure that adequate numbers of viable organisms survive the concentration, freeze-drying or drying process needed to prepare a stable commercial product" (1984) J Appld Nutri.36. 125 -153.

Probiotic prescribing and care of the intestinal flora in health and disease fits particularly into concepts of Reckeweg's Homotoxicology, Pischinger's Biological matrix and Dubois/Vincent "Terraine", or Biological Terrain (the 'body soil'), as also the aims of Naturopathy, e.g. to help the body in its self-repairing efforts; in treating people not disease; in removing the cause of disease not merely its symptoms; in curing the disease not just postponing it.

The use of Probiotics in therapy must be in accord with the "Philosophy of Natural Therapeutics" as expounded by Henry Lindlahr (1919), i.e. the natural therapeutic approach maintains that the constant effort of the body's life force is always in the direction of self-cleansing, self-repairing and positive health. The philosophy maintains that even acute disease is a manifestation of the body's efforts in the direction of self-cure. Disease, or downgraded health, may be eliminated only by removing from the system the real cause, and by raising the body's general vitality, so that its natural and inherent ability to sustain health is allowed to dominate. Natural therapeutic philosophy also maintains that chronic diseases are frequently the results of mistaken efforts to cure, or attempted suppression of the physiological efforts of the body to cleanse itself. Such philosophy certainly could be considered a background to nutritional therapy, probiotic therapy and indeed Anti-Homotoxic therapy. Lindlahr goes on to state "Every acute disease is the result of a healing effort of nature" (Reckeweg concurs in his Theory of Homotoxicology), i.e. disease symptomatology is an action made by the body as a result of a cause and effect relationship - echoes of antibiotic and probiotic actions here.

Nearly every action of modern day, "Western", industrialised, urbanised, techno-econo-politico living causes disharmony in the physical, mental, emotional and moral planes of our existence. Thus to understand the direction and purpose of the disease process, it is necessary to look at the causes of disease from a naturopathic, rather than classical pathological viewpoint, i.e. more holistically:

a) Accumulation of toxic material in the body, the result of improper diet, alcohol, coffee, tobacco, "social" drugs with resultant oxygen/nitrogen species free radical activity, combined with poor blood and lymph circulation due to low levels of stimulatory physical activity and hence poor elimination, is crucial here. Thus, accumulations within the cells, especially toxic elements, ultimately lead to changes of structure, function and immunological competence, and hence reduced resistance to disease.

b) Incorrect or unbalanced diets, with resultant reduced vitality, essential nutrient deficiency, toxaemia, poor elimination (due to lack of dietary fibre, see previously). Our diet, compared with that of our ancestors (composed of whole grains, nuts, raw fruits, fresh vegetables, simple proteins occasionally and pure water), is now made up of refined carbohydrates, de-vitalised grains, highly salted, frozen, canned or poisoned fruits, 'limp, long delay' vegetables, complex proteins poisoned by drugs and chemicals and polluted 'recycled' water. The trend to food refining and modification today leads to an unbalanced, low fibre, unnatural diet with reduced nutrient value of the food. High-yield fertilisers and their over use, affects the natural balance and vitality of the soil, resulting in nutrient (especially mineral) inferior and deficient food. Pesticides, herbicides and additives (preservatives), place a burden on the body to detoxify - this toxic burden directly and indirectly affects the intestinal micro-ecology.

c) Physical/Body Mechanic Dysfunction - resulting from lack of demanding physical exercise for the body to which end it was designed and evolved, today does little to promote optimum functioning, indeed the opposite. Thus, poor muscle tone predisposes to accident and injury, and interferes with blood and lymph circulation, and poor posture causes reduction in internal organ optimum function; with toxic accumulation and hence disease; especially due to reduced drainage and toxic elimination.

d) Stress/Mental/Emotional Disturbances - upset blood flow, hormone balance, metabolic biochemistry directly and via psycho-neuro-endocrine-immunological linkages. Such in the long term result in lowered vitality and susceptibility to disease. The intestinal flora may be primarily (radiation, infra sound - low frequency, fear, anxiety, anger, resentment), or secondarily (chemical exotoxins, antigens (allergens), pollutants, drugs - especially antibiotics, cortisone - food additives, etc.) affected. Electromagnetic sensitivity and so-called 'sick-building' syndrome and similar environmental/climatic effects (positive ions - the Fohne in Swiss - neuro-vegatitive dystony is created, which theoretically via A.N.S links may affect the micro flora), M.E. and the 'fibromyalgia syndrome' may develop.

So, on to chronic disease which Lindlahr defines thus:

"A condition of the organism in which lowered vibration (vitality), due to accumulation of waste materials and poisons (toxins), with the consequent destruction of vital parts and organs, has progressed to such an extent that nature's constructive and healing forces are no longer able to act against the disease conditions by acute corrective efforts (healing crisis)."

You, the reader, may note shades of Homotoxicology Reckeweg, Pischinger, Smidt and Vincent here.

Many distinct pointers are made above to food influences. It is most important to "prescribe" in parallel to Probiotics - a system of optimum nutrition. Such a principle in depth is beyond the scope of this short book (The EAB-MS Course 'Food and Health" leading to the Royal Society of Health Certificate is recommended for practitioners using Probiotics). Basically, live yoghurt and other cultured milk products are obvious dietary factors. 'Functional foods" - such as Chlorella, Spirulina (known by references to enhance the micro flora), and Aloe Vera are obvious supplements, which the author believes are paramount in stimulating the bowel flora - the cell walls of Chlorella providing an enhanced dietary fibre matrix for microflora growth as well as a total nutrient supplement for the person and his intestinal flora alike - garlic, biotin and caprylic acid are useful adjuncts.

The recommended associate diet is one that is rich in complex carbohydrates such as fresh vegetables, pulses, seeds, nuts and whole grains (wheat, oats, brown rice, millet, etc). In addition, soy products (it would be interesting to know if genetically engineered Soya has lost its benefit in this respect - does anyone out there know of any relevant research in this sphere?). Emphasis is therefore on a macrobiotic or lacto-vegetarian diet (but fish, poultry - minus skin, and perhaps game are acceptable, whereas pig products are most detrimental - see Reckeweg). Miso and Tofu, as fermented soy products, are most valuable. Quorn, bean and other sproutings, watercress, organic vegetables and natural home-made juices are recommended. Probiotics should be taken with natural mineral water (NOT chlorinated water). Kombucha tea is recommended but synthetic compound vitamin and mineral supplements are not, though natural Vitamin C could be useful in early stages. However most vitamin and mineral supplements are contained in sufficient doses in whole foods such as Spirulina, Chlorella and Aloe Vera.

It is not only in humans but also in animals (especially horses), that supplementation of Probiotics is valuable. Miss Deborah M Lucas BSc. MSc. (Equine Science), refers to the horse as a trickle feeder with a digestive system designed to contend with small, very frequent meals of high fibres, low soluble carbohydrate foods. The anatomy of the equine digestive tract reflects this emphasis, with the large intestine - the area for fibre digestion containing a vast microbial population - making up about 63% of the total volume of the gut. Thus, the microbial population is of vital significance in digesting fibre, and in the production of certain vitamins. However, the stresses imposed upon the modern horse often predispose this microbial population to severe disruption. This results at best in reduced efficiency of digestion, and at worst allow the invasion and establishment of undesirable and pathogenic bacteria. Miss Lucas considers that the inclusion of probiotics in the diet of horses subjected to stress - racehorses, brood mares, youngstock and competition horses - enables the microbial population to be maintained and replenished to ensure that well being and performance is not affected. Thus, there is a prophylactic (immune system enhancement), and therapeutic use (especially in equine flu etc.) have shown to improve performance and condition in almost all categories of horses.

In the USA, (survey in 1985), 225 veterinarians showed that 60% of them either prescribed or dispensed probiotics for farm animals or horses in the preceding 18 months. Their use in order of importance was: newly born foals, dairy replacement calves, growing adult horses, lactating dairy cows, brought-in beef cattle, newly born calves, weaned calves, pets and other animals. Mr Bruce Manley, Manager of the Bacton Stud, has stated that excellent results were obtained following the use of probiotics in brood mares and their foals at studs and when used in competitive animals. Results showed that when compared with controls, the growth rates and general condition of the 'probiotic' animals was improved by around 20% as a consequence of better food utilisation. Scour in the young foals was drastically reduced, respiratory problems were found to be more easily controlled by antibiotics, mares showed less signs of stress during parturition, and better conception rates at first oestrus after foaling. In addition, probiotic fed mares produced a good bloom on their coats, showing a distinct improvement over controls. In a series of around 500 horses in training on the flat in 1987, plus 20 event horses, probiotic fed horses consistently achieved better results and won more races than previously. Form was maintained longer too. Several major Group Races were won by horses being fed probiotics regularly and the horse which finished second in the major 3-Day Event at Burghley was being fed probiotics.

In A. Pischinger MD "Matrix and Matrix Regulation" 1991, edited by Prof Hartmut Heine PhD, it states that the intestinal flora relationships and intestinal function is important for the success of regulatory therapy. In chronic diseases the intestinal flora relationships are normal in only 2.5% of the patients; in 97.5% the balance is more or less severe. He states, "it should never be forgotten that gastric acid deficiency and ferment insufficiency, for example after disease of the liver and pancreas, have to be treated at the same time or order to prevent a general recurrence of the imbalance of the flora".

In terms of 'disturbance field theory' the largest disturbance area is often the intestinal system, and that diseases (allergies, eczema, etc.), resist therapy until the disturbances and their general effects, i.e. the intestinal flora and function, are cured. It was only possible to establish disturbances of the intestinal flora with precision after 1982. Prof J THURNER in Vienna 1982-87 carried out about 1700 stool cultures and showed a totally varying picture in intestinal micro-organism aberrations, with consequences for the total defence process.

Primary intestinal flora aberrations arise from a variety of causes:

a) Gastric Acid deficiency
b) Intestinal Infections - salmonellosis, shigeliosis, parasitosis especially Gardiasis - Lambliosis in Europe/Russia.
c) Antibacterial therapy, antibiotics, sulphonamides, umidazole, etc.
d) Fungal/yeast infestation - to which I would add -
e) Radiation, EMF, Sound Vibration (Infrasound in particular).

Secondary disturbances occur in severe disturbances of the total defence performance - in cancer patients after immuno-suppressive therapy, in the late stages of inflammatory diseases, (e.g. TB, PCP and MS), and in inherited and acquired immune deficiency. There are many types of intestinal flora disturbance - in 46% of the investigations there is a complete deficiency of Escherichia coli (eubiotic not pathogenic), and in 41.7% a complete deficiency of the lactic-acid forming Lactobacillus acidophilus and Bacterium bifidum. E-coli produces, amongst other substances, Pischinger's Monocyte factor, which is important for the activation of the function of Peyer's plaques and the intestinal lymph nodes (formation of lymphocyte factor). In 61.2% of all cultures, fungi are found, mainly Candida albicans, but also Candida spec., Parapsilosis, Trichosporum spec., Geotrictium spec., Rhodotorula spec., Torulopsis spec., Tropicalis spec., the pathogenic effect depends on the quantity present, i.e. above 10 organisms/g of stool. Such fungal entities above set off disturbances that are graded as toxic: especially their metabolic products and inflammatory (colitic) signs and symptoms develop as well as the intestinal flora upsets.

At this stage it is important to emphasise that PRIOR to any Probiotic usage, it is ESSENTIAL to organise a faecal stool parasitology examination. This is particularly to EXCLUDE the very common protozoa - Giardia lamblia - 32% were found positive in one North European survey. It is becoming more ubiquitous and this may be due to warmer winters; and it occurs particularly if there is sub-acidity or an-acidity of the stomach, and it viciously competes for nutrients required by the flora (and the person), and may result in essential mineral deficiencies, leading to disturbance of the defence cycles. It is important to realise that any disturbance in the balance of the intestinal flora lead to important disturbances of defence performance capacity (immune system competency), hence probiotics can be considered IMMUNO- MODULATORS in respect of:

a) Absorption disturbances (vitamins, minerals, trace elements).
b) Toxins (products of imbalance, decomposition, fungi).
c) Blockade of abdominal lymph apparatus by toxins.

Thus, the intestinal tract can become an extensive disturbance field for the regulatory system, and creates stresses for the ground system through toxins and mineral deficiencies. So total nutrient functional foods, i.e. Spirulina, Chlorella, Aloe must be given as an adjunct to Probiotics.

Part I : The Intestine in Health - Overview

1.1 The Anatomy and Physiology

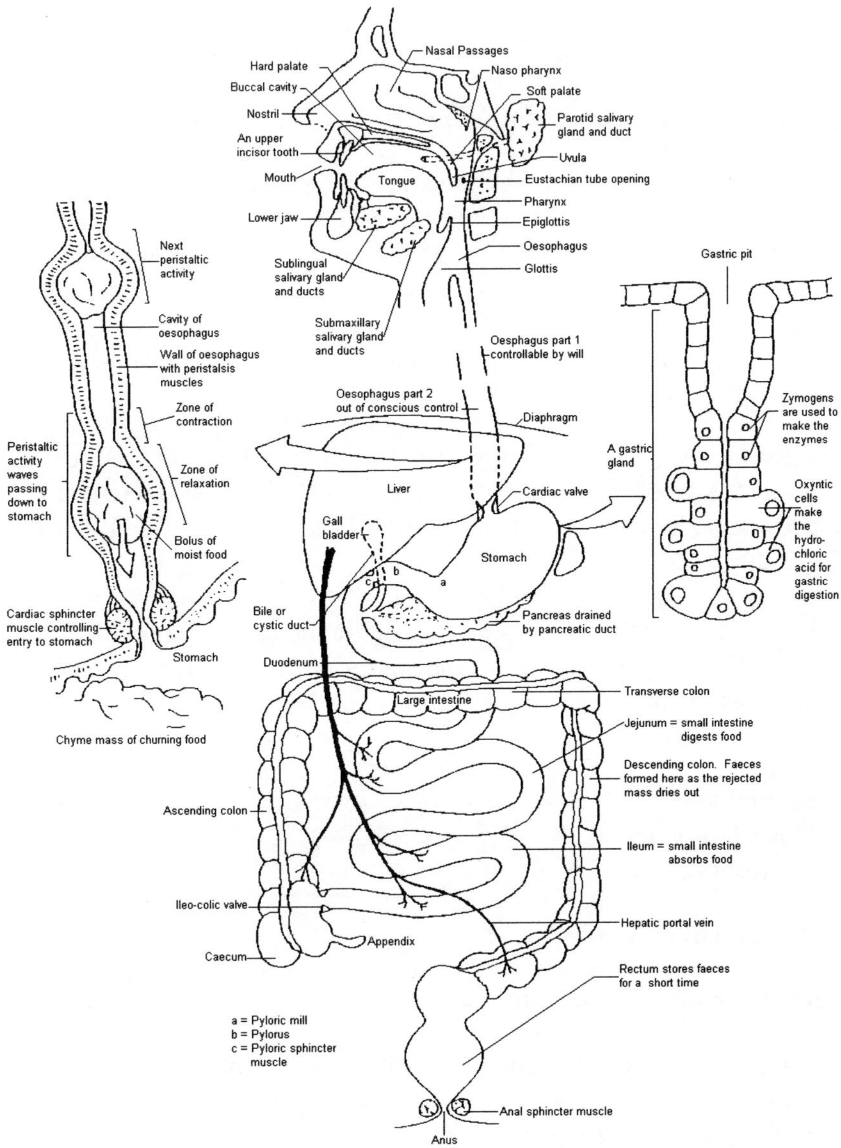

1.1.1 The digestive system aids the correct functioning of the cell by ensuring that the body is provided with the biological molecules necessary to maintain cellular metabolism and cellular homeostasis.

Food intake is regulated by the hypothalamus, where there are 2 centres for the regulation of food intake:

a) Hunger Centre - constantly active unless inhibited by activity from:

b) Satiety (cessation of feeding) Centre.

There are innumerable theories as to how food intake is regulated in human beings, and many factors involved. The present concept is that of gastrointestinal 'stretch receptors' of the stomach and duodenum. These receptors have afferent sensory input to the centres, and are balanced in 'firing' - thus the satiety centre during and immediately after feeding produces sufficiently powerful output to inhibit the hunger centre and hence causes the cessation of food intake.

Detailed anatomy and histology of the gastrointestinal tract is beyond the scope of this book - readers are referred to "Physiology and Anatomy - a homeostatic approach" by Clancy and McVicar Arnold 1995 ISBN 0-340-63190-2.

Suffice it to look at the diagrams, especially the cross section of duodenum and note the 4 layers, which are present to a greater or lesser extent from oesophagus to anus i.e.

1/ Mucosa
2/ Submucosa
3/ Muscularis external
4/ Sclerosa/Ventitia

1.1.2 Control of Salivation

There are 3 main pairs of salivary glands:

1/ Parotid - specific cells producing water and enzymes
2/ Submandibular - as above, but with greater mucus content
3/ Sublingual - mucus + +, very little enzyme

Water is 90 - 95% in the saliva, the rest being mucin mainly, then enzymes and solutes, thus:

1/ Mucin forming mucus with water - lubricating action
2/ Lysozymes - destroy bacteria
3/ Salivary Amylase - initiates carbohydrate digestion
4/ Antibodies - gammaglobulins, immunoglobulin A
5/ Urea, albumin
6/ Ions - sodium, potassium, bicarbonates, chlorides (activate salivary amylase phosphates)
7/ Lingual lipase which acts on triglycerides

The autonomic nervous system controls salivation, mainly via the brain stem parasympathetic neurones. Dehydration homeostatically stimulates the thirst centre, yet in times of high stress, the sympathetic response produces dryness of the mouth and produces thick sticky saliva - a homeostatic type response.

Conditioned 'Pavlovian' type responses, upon encounter with kitchen smells, or meal anticipation, result in salivary flow, such responses being the result of conditioned memory responses, thus saliva is ready for the food intake.

The Alimentary Canal function is regulated both by nerve and hormone co-ordination.

The mouth area functions under the trigeminal, facial and glossopharyngeal nerves, while the swallowing reflex is a function of the facial nerve and the vagus nerve. A combination of action of the facial/mesenteric and Auerbachs plexus controls and co-ordinates peristalsis in the oesophagus.

1.1.3 The movement of food from the mouth into the stomach is achieved by the act of deglutition of the pharynx and peristalsis of the oesophagus.

The stomach has glands containing 5 cell types:

a) Mucous surface cells - secrete mucus
b) Mucous neck cell - secretes mucus
c) Parietal cells - secreting hydrochloric acid and intrinsic factor
d) Zymogenic cells - secrete pepsinogen and gastric lipase
e) Entero-endocrine cell (G cell) - secretes gastrin

Both neural and hormonal mechanisms act to control the secretion of gastric juice and the contractions of smooth muscle in the stomach wall.

1.1.4 Small Intestine - where major events of digestion and absorption take place. The villi and microvilli increase the surface area, and there are 4 types of cell:

a) Absorptive Cell - digests and absorbs nutrients
b) Goblet Cell - secretes mucus
c) Entero - endocrine Cell - secretes secretin, cholecystokinin (CCK) also known as glucose - dependent insulinotropic peptide
d) Paneth Cell - secretes lysozyme and is capable of phagocytosis an so is most relevant in the picture of micro-ecology of the gut, and so may have a role in regulating the microbial population.

The inner layer of the villi (lamina propria) of the small intestine has much mucosa-associated lymphoid tissue (MALT) which also extends to the submucosal area (see later). There are also solitary lymphatic nodules, mainly at the distal end. Aggregated lymphatic follicles (Peyer's patches) are scattered throughout the ileum. They have a vital role in the immune system function.

1.1.5 The Large Intestine - the overall functions:

a) Completion of absorption
b) Production of certain vitamins
c) Formation of faeces
d) Expulsion of faeces

Certain 'digestive' functions of the large intestine depend on 2 key factors:

a) the extent and nature of the dietary fibre (see later)
b) the extent and nature of the indigenous microflora of the lumen of the large intestine

If all in good order then synthesis of certain B vitamins and vitamin K takes place, while the mucosa seeks to maintain water balance, absorb certain mineral ions, and the synthesised vitamins. Certainly, as we shall see later, the well functioning intestinal flora plays an important role in immune system function and effectiveness.

Part 1.2. - Co-ordination and Control of the Alimentary Canal - for total understanding, this subject needs detailed study, especially of the pathways of the Autonomic Nervous System (Sympathetic and Parasympathetic) and the Hormonal System.

1.2.1 The basic organisation of the nervous systems involved in the control and co-ordination of the digestive system:

A. Enteric nervous system (ENS) - mediating local reflexes.
B. Links between the ENS and ganglia outside the digestive system - mediating ganglionic reflexes.
C. Links between the central nervous system and the ganglia and the ENS - mediating spinal and brain stem reflexes.
D. The Autonomic Nervous System. N.B. Sympathetic and para-sympathetic have opposing effects on organs that receive dual innervation.

1/ Mucous membrane of nose and palate
a) Sympathetic via superior cervical ganglion (TI)
b) Parasympathetic via pterygopalatine ganglion (VII cranio-sacral)

2/ Sublingual and Submandibular Glands
a) Sympathetic as above
b) Parasympathetic via submandibular ganglion (VII cranio-sacral)

3/ Parotid Gland
Parasympathetic only via the otic ganglion (IX cranio-sacral)

4/ Stomach
a) Sympathetic via coeliac ganglion (T VI to T XII)
b) Parasympathetic directly (from Vagus X cranio-sacral)

5/ Liver, Gall Bladder, Bile ducts, Pancreas, Spleen
a) Sympathetic via coeliac ganglion
b) Parasympathetic directly (from Vagus X cranio-sacral)

6/ Small Intestine, Ascending, Transverse and Descending Colons
a) Sympathetic via superior mesenteric ganglia and inferior mesenteric ganglion (descending and sigmoid colon)
b) Parasympathetic via direct innervation from Vagus X except ascending and sigmoid colon via pelvic splanchnic nerve (S2)

This may seem unnecessarily detailed to the reader, but knowledge of this balanced control is important to the understanding of alimentary canal structure and function.

If not clear refer to the following further reading:

1) Physiology and Anatomy - a basis for nursing and health care - elementary overall picture, RUTISHAUSER. Churchill Livingstone.
2) Principles of Anatomy and Physiology 9th edition 2000 - invaluable but advanced, TORTORA & GRABOWSKI. John Wiley & Sons Inc.

1.2.2 The Basic Organisation of the Hormonal Systems

A. Major Hormones

1) Gastrin - promotes secretion and motility, constricts lower oesophageal sphincter, relaxes pyloric sphincter and ileocaecal sphincter.

2) Gastric inhibitory peptide (GIP) - stimulates release of insulin, inhibits secretion of gastric juice, slows gastric emptying.
3) Secretin - stimulates pancreatic juice HCO_3 - inhibits secretion of gastric juice, and enhances effects of CCK.

4) Cholecystokinin (CCK) - stimulates secretion of pancreatic juice, bile ejection. Satiety sometimes CCK-PZ - also inhibits gastric emptying, and promotes growth and maintenance of the pancreas and enhances effects of secretin.

B. 10 Minor Hormones - some with 'neuro -transmitter'type action:

a) Motilin)
b) Substance P) Stimulate motility of intestines
c) Bombesin)
d) Vaso-active intestinal polypeptide (VIP) - ions, water - secretion stimulated & gastric acid inhibitor
e) Gastrin-releasing peptide (GRP) - stimulates gastrin release
f) Somatostatin - inhibits gastric release
g) Serotonin (5-HT) - various function, may be implicated in 'satiety'& mood control, induction of sleep
h) Encephalins- relaxants, inhibit pain impulses by suppressing release of substance P
i) Neurotensin - functions not clear

Substance P is known to enhance perception of pain (neuropeptide).

All of these have direct and indirect influences and effect on the intestinal flora/probiotics.

Part 1.3 - Immunological Aspects - Mucosal and Floral

Mucosal surfaces are in contact with the host and the environment from which they are exposed to antigens i.e. food antigens, and pathogenic micro-organisms. The gut associated lymphoid system (GALT) comprises the largest part of the immune system, and is in intimate contact with the normal intestinal microflora. Similarly, there is mucosal-associated lymphoid tissue (MALT) in the nasopharyngeal and bronchial regions, urogenital areas etc.

GALT is present as Peyer's patches, the caecal appendix, the mesenter lymph nodes (MLN) and some solitary lymphoid nodules. The epithelium overlying the Peyer's patches contains M cells. Such are important in mucosal immunity, and much more research is required on them. Basically, they seem to act as specialised epithelial cells, which transport antigen from the gut lumen to the underlying lymphoid cells, presumably by some form of phagocytosis. Once in the Peyer's patches these bacteria and bacterial antigens are destroyed and the antigens are presented to B and T lymphocytic cells. These then seem to circulate in the blood stream for a while and then resettle in the lamina propria of the gut wall. Meantime some redevelop into more plasma cell-like bodies and produce secretory IgA by a complex process predominantly, but in certain situations IgG and IgM antibodies also seem to be produced.

It is only possible to be aware of normal healthy states in respect of this mucosal immunity facility, by studying and observing what happens in disease states.

Thus, different, randomised, controlled clinical trials have demonstrated that Lactobacillus rhamnosus GC, together with L.casei DN 114001 (LC) is effective in the treatment of gastro-enteritis, especially in the case of infant rotavirus diarrhoea. Also, in situations of gastrointestinal inflammation, such as during ulcerative colitis and Crohn's disease the adaptive cytokine network seems to be invoked and may in turn create chronic states. Lactobacilli, probably via immuno-modulation, seem to alleviate such states.

There also seems to be other 'links and associations' to upset intestinal floral balance, affecting mucosal and systemic immunity especially in areas of autoimmune conditions such as Ankylosing spondylitis, rheumatoid arthritis, myasthenia gravis, lupus erythematosis, and some forms of motor neurone disease. Research at Kings College Hospital, London, indicates that certain types of different bacteria have certain tissue-type connotations i.e. Klebsiella relative to B27 tissue type and hence the immune system 'mistakes' own body tissue and induces self -attack resulting in these autoimmune states. The indigenous or supplemented Lactobacteria tend to result in recovery or arrest of autoimmune states; and hence it is logical to assume that they act prophylactically.

Equally, there seems to be a close relationship and influence on the MALT as vice versa. Thus, it appears that the normal flora seems to be able to regulate the immune reactivity of the whole organism, but this seems to depend on bacterial group types. Thus, the microflora can be deemed to have a modulating effect on the intestinal immune system; and that allergy (hypersensitivity) and autoimmune phenomena maybe related to disturbances in intestinal colonisation - a state known as dysbiosis. A weak and slow antibody response is characteristic of food antigens, but under certain circumstances the functions between epithelial cells become weak and a condition of 'leaky -gut syndrome' ensues.

Part 1.4 - Psycho-Neuro-Endocrine-Immunological Aspects (PNEI)

As the consideration of antigen effects in 1.3, PNEI will be considered briefly, mainly in relation to stress and stressors (often toxins).

Stress, according to P.H.Black, is " a state of disharmony or threatened homeostasis provoked by a psychological, environmental or physiological stressor". Such cause response via the hypothalmic-pituitary-adrenal (HPA) axis, and which response is integrated and affects the sympathetic nervous and endocrine systems, with inbuilt positive and negative active regulatory interactions. Inevitably, such affect GALT and in turn the gut microflora as also vice versa.

Neurotransmitters and circulating neuropeptides are generated and form the basis of the stress response at general and local levels, and undoubtedly affect the gut microflora; as a host of immune and inflammatory mediators are released with multifactorial effects; depending on the stressor stimulus; and the degree of psychological adaptation ability exhibited by the individual stimulated.

Briefly, in addition to other bodily effects, there can develop actual damage to the gut lining, resulting in inflammation, local minute haemorrhages and often local swelling. Such changes have a variety of effects on the state of the microflora, mainly via locally produced toxins and often putrefactive products. These, in many situations, especially where the lining of the

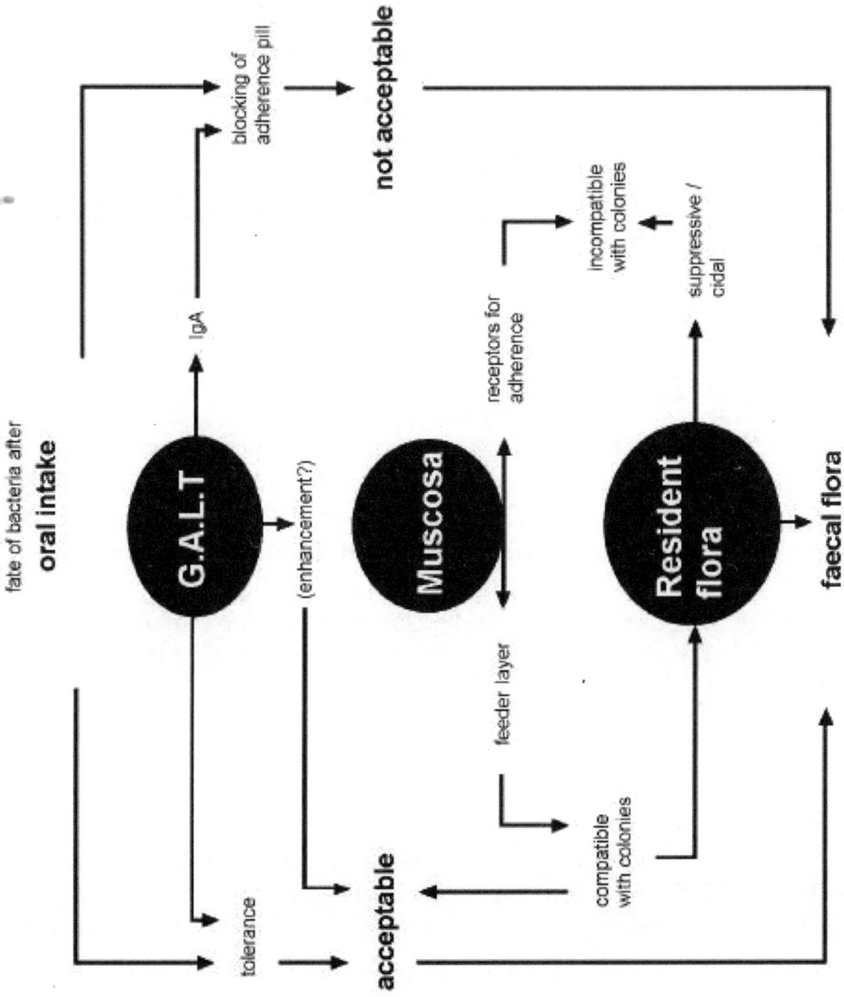
fate of bacteria after
oral intake
G.A.L.T
IgA
blocking of
adherence pili
not acceptable
(enhancement?)
tolerance
acceptable
Muscosa
receptors for
adherence
feeder layer
incompatible
with colonies
suppressive /
cidal
compatible
with colonies
Resident
flora
faecal flora

mucosa is damaged, can 'leak' into the blood stream. Allergic and inflammatory responses are thereby induced.

A healthy intestinal microflora where balance is good tends to prevent such stress effects, which induce changes and reduce lactobacilli and bifidobacteria and allow 'invaders'. Obviously, supplementation must be beneficial.

Part 1.5 - Role of Dietary Fibre

Fibre can be considered an essential dietary substance, which is as important as any other essential nutrient; though not a nutrient in its own right. If ingested daily in sufficient variety, quality and quantity, then it has been found to lead to improvement of health and well-being, while also preventing certain degenerative, metabolic, autoimmune and cancerous conditions.

The W.H.O recommends an increase in daily fibre intake, especially for the majority consuming the typical diet in urbanised technologically dominated so-called Western societies. The typical diet of this populace consists of high intake of refined carbohydrate, saturated fat and animal protein; which provides on average about 20 grammes of dietary fibre daily. The W.H.O recommends that dietary fibre intake is best in the form of fresh fruit and vegetables, whole grains, beans and lentils, rather than bran or other supplements.

In 1980 the Royal College of Physicians UK produced a report, "Medical aspects of Dietary Fibre". It states, "in so far as giving fibre may lead to smaller intake of refined carbohydrate, and other energy rich nutrients, it may be expected to improve dental health, and to control obesity, with a possible preventive action on the concomitants of obesity, such as gallstones, non-insulin dependent diabetes mellitus, (NIDDM), ischaemic heart disease and cancer of the colon". Regrettably, much of this message has gone unheeded, in spite of the 'medical establishment' rationality accorded to the necessity for dietary fibre indicated by the report.

Fibre was formerly regarded as an injurious gastrointestinal irritant and was termed roughage - this is now considered an old fashioned terms and should not be used. As Arrow states in Human Nutrition and Dietetics, "a major barrier to progress in understanding dietary fibre and its role has been the lack of an agreed chemical definition of dietary fibre. This has delayed the development of accurate methods for its measurement and

"Defence" of the mucosal surfaces

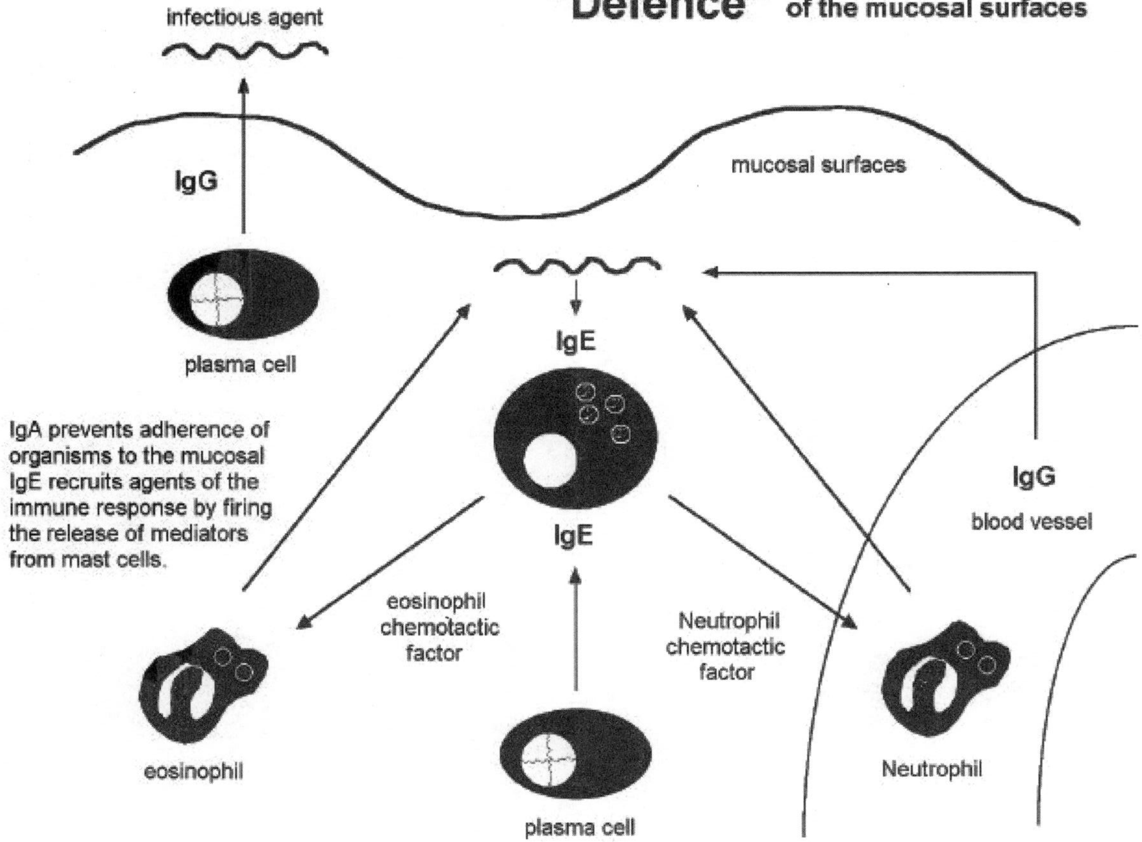

resulted in the misinterpretation of studies of dietary fibre in man" (English).

Thus, as will be outlined below, the concept of dietary fibre, from its first use by Hipsley, (1953), to the present parlance of non-starch polysaccharides, (NSP), in plant food, has changed over the years. Trowell in 1972 defined dietary fibre as the skeletal remains of plant cells that are resistant to digestion by the enzymes of man.

So, the dietary fibre hypothesis of Burkitt and Trowell was formulated in two basic components:

1) a diet rich in foods which contain plant cell walls, (i.e. whole grains, legumes, fruits and vegetables), is protective against a wide variety of diseases, in particular those that are prevalent in western industrialised society.

2) a diet providing a low intake of plant cell walls is a causative factor in the aetiology of these diseases and provides conditions under which other aetiological factors are more active.

Burkitt, subsequent to in-depth epidemiological studies, produced a sequence of events thus:

Stage I - the more primitive diet of plant eaters which contains large amounts of unprocessed starch staples, in such situations there are few cases of diseases associated with low "fibre" diet, (see later).

Stage II - early so-called 'Westernisation' of diet, but obesity and diabetes occur in privileged groups, and those spending time abroad from local diet.

Stage III - moderate 'Westernisation' of diet, where in addition to stage II problems, cases of constipation, haemorrhoids, varicose veins and appendicitis are common.

Stage IV- full 'Westernisation' where ischaemic heart disease, diverticular disease, hiatus hernia and cancer become common.

Interestingly enough, Hippocrates disapproved of "new white breads", and Galen, a father physician, in his book "Faculties or Powers of Ailments" devoted 71 chapters on "fibre foods", i.e. fruits and vegetables, which he advocated. Certainly, also Ayurvedic preventative medicine and dietary concepts of "Foods that Heal" are in accord.

In respect of colonic function relevant to intestinal microbiology and clinical ecology, dietary fibre plays a role in providing a medium and a matrix (or stroma), for the growth of the desirable and health promoting indigenous bacteria.

Thus, it is able to classify diseased associated with low fibre diet:

1) METABOLIC - obesity, diabetes, gall stones, gout, multiple sclerosis, senile osteoporosis, pernicious anaemia, PMS.

2) CARDIOVASCULAR - high cholesterol, atherosclerosis, ischaemic heart disease, hypertension, cerebro-vascular disease, varicose veins, haemorrhoids, deep vein thrombosis, pulmonary embolism.

3) COLONIC - constipation, appendicitis, diverticulitis, diverticulosis, Crohn's Disease, ulcerative colitis, haemorrhoids, polyps, irritable bowel syndrome (?), cancer of the large bowel. Dysbiosis + effects.

4) OTHER - dental caries, autoimmune disorders, skin disorders.

A detailed and exact study of dietary fibre or NSP, if you wish to be 'at the leading edge', is an essential knowledge module for probiotic prescribers, for the fibre matrix is the 'key' to intestinal function, neural and hormonal, while also the functional state of probiotic endeavour. If the NSP intake is insufficient, then probiotic supplementation effect becomes diminished. Equally, the author, in accord with published work, believes parallel functional food, i.e. Chlorella, (with cell wall NSP matrix), or Spirulina, (known to enhance intestinal flora and growth and function), or Aloe Vera, (acts similarly), is essential to probiotic usage.

Also, internal 'prescription' of garlic, which exerts antibacterial, anti -viral and anti-fungal/anti-yeast activity is PARAMOUNT, (Physiotherapy Res. 1991:5 154-8). Internal use of garlic may inhibit growth of yeast organisms, (esp. Candida species), and increase resistance to yeast infections. For persons with no aversion to the odour, one whole clove of raw garlic can be chewed or used in food daily, possible as pre-prepared granules. Otherwise, odour-controlled, enteric-coated tablets, or garlic powder - around 300mgs garlic powder providing 4g of alliin, the proactive substance together with the enzyme allinase. Product monitoring and control of the various preparations available must be ensured.

The term NSP - non-starch polysaccharides - has replaced the former term 'dietary fibre', and as such gives the best index (in f ood labelling), of plant cell-wall polysaccharides - basically the dietary intake of carbohydrate material that is not composed of sugar and starches. NSP can be divided into two types - water-soluble NSP, i.e. pectins, gums, mucilates and algal polysaccharides, and insoluble NSP, i.e. cellulose, hemi-celluloses and lignins.

The composition of the plant cell wall varies according to the species of plant. Typically the dry cell wall contains 35% cellulose, 45% non-cellulose polysaccharides, 17% lignins, (not included in the analytical definition of dietary fibre (Englyst et al 1987), 3% protein and 2% ash. The cell wall contains cellulose molecules organised in discrete fibrils, surround by the matrix polysaccharides and lignin.. The cellulose fibrils are surrounded by a sheath of xylo-glucans, which are hydrogen-bonded to the cellulose. The other non-cellulose polysaccharides are covalently linked with the xyloglucan, with the cell wall protein and with one other, so that the matrix is in effect a highly ordered super-molecule. It is thought that this matrix configuration is important in forming the loculi for micro flora to reproduce: especially the network of cellulose fibrils.

1) **Cellulose** - high molecular - weight linear polymer of up to 10,000 units linked *B*(1-4)D glucan. Cellulose is insoluble in water, but has an ability to bind water: thus increasing faecal size and weight and hence promoting regular bowel movements. So constipation is reduced and relieved. Certainly it appears that Chlorella, by virtue of the 'broken' cellulose cell walls, can provide not only a niche matrix for "friendly" bacteria to reproduce, it can provide the necessary 'in house' nutrients, according to Japanese research, to attain the "enhanced intestinal tract optimum facility objective" in this respect.

Humans cannot digest cellulose, though the bacteria of the large intestine undertake a fermentation process which results in partial degradation of the cellulose, which leads to the production of short chain fatty acids, together with gases and indeed energy for the colon and possibly for the liver. The short chain fatty acids (SCFAs), i.e. acetic, propionic and butyric acids, have various differing roles, i.e. butyrate is energy source for colonic cells, and may also exert anti-cancer properties, whereas proprinate and acetate are more concerned at liver level. A diet high in dietary fibre promotes the growth of acid loving bacteria because of the increasing synthesis of SCFAs, which result in a reduction of colon pH, i.e. increased acidity.

All dietary fibre, not just cellulose, plays a vital role in colonic function, especially in respect of the bacterial flora in the colon. First of all it plays a role in providing a medium for the growth of the desirable and health promoting acid-loving bacteria by means of producing SCFAs mentioned above, together with a general acid environment. Such happens around the matrix or stroma produced by the dietary fibre, providing facility for the lacto, and other 'friendly' bacilli to synthesise various B group vitamins and foliate coenzymes.

Alongside, there is a reduction of the activity of faecal nitro-reductase and azo-reductase. These, especially the latter, reputedly catalyse the conversion of pro carcinogens into carcinogens (cancer producing agents).

Deconfiguration of bile acids in the intestinal tract is enhanced by adequate fibre intake, and an anto-cholesteraemic effect has been recorded.

The B group vitamins synthesised are niacin (reduces cholesterol), pantothenic acid (vitamin B5), pyridoxines (vitamin B6), cyanocobolamine (vitamin B12) and Folic Acid.

Furthermore, Lactobacillus casei can inhibit Salmonella, Vibrio species, undesirable E.coli species, and Staphylococcus' aureus species (possibly including the multiple resistant varieties) - all of which can cause 'food' poisoning. Equally, L.bifidus is antagonistic against E.coli species, Shigella species (causing dysentery), and Salmonella typhimurium (typhoid). Numerous workers have reported isolating natural antibiotics, i.e. Acidophillin from L.acidophilus, bulgarican or bulgaricin from L.bulgaricus, together with lactolin and lactocidin. In addition, several species of Lactobacilli produce hydrogen peroxide which inhibits Staph.Aureus, Pseudonomas and certain disease producing strains of E.coli, (which can synthesise ethiomine and nitrosamine, from nitrates and nitrites, both of which are known to be potentially carcinogenic).

From these factors there has developed the rationale of prescribing Acidophilus strains, (especially DDSI), in cases of gastro-enteritis, especially in infants, as perhaps also in the therapeutic technique of colonic irrigation with acidophilus implants (such are also the techniques of ancient Ayurvedic medical using 'curd' fermented milk).

The dietary fibre may also provide a suitable environment to enhance the 'productivity' of the Peyer's patches in the intestine (lymphoid tissue, producing B. Lymphocytes - immune system factors). Fibre also prevents the absorption of toxic heavy metal and organic toxins from metabolic products, including trans-fatty acids and triglycerides. This may well explain the therapeutic value of high fibre, low refined carbohydrate low saturate fat with lactobacillus supplementation in the management of acne vulgaris cases.

2) **Hemicelluloses** are also plant polysaccharides, containing mainly pentose sugars, hexose, xylose, arabinose, both of the latter in the form of xylans, together with polymerised acidic sugars such as galacturonic and glucoronic acids. The colon does act to degrade these substances, they can and do absorb water and are a source of short chain fatty acids.

3) **Lignins** are present in the woody tissue of vegetables, and are strictly polysaccharides, and they are totally indigestible. Chemically they are aromatic polymers composed mainly of cinnamic acid, cinnamyl alcohol, propenyl benzene and allylbenzene precursor units. The gut flora produce enterolactone and enterodiol. Lignins by virtue of their alcohol content also exhibit antibiotic; anti-fungal and antiviral activity.

4) **Pectin and Pectin-Like Substances** - also originate from plant cell walls, and are basically polymers of galacturonic acid. They are not fibrous, and are water soluble and digestible, and can be found in orange rind, apple peel and onion skins. They reduce the rate of gastric emptying, thereby slowing the rate at which carbohydrates (especially sugars) are digested and absorbed. They also lower cholesterol levels by binding it, together with bile salts and enhancing excretion.

5) **Mucilages** - these are mixed non-fibrous polymers of arabinose, xylose, mannose, glucoronic and galacturonic acids. They are generally found within the endosperm of plant seeds. They originate from beans (legumes), and exhibit water soluble and digestible properties. They act to induce satiety, prevent excess energy intake, slow down gastric emptying and sugar uptake, and reduce serum cholesterol levels, possibly by increasing excretion of bile salts and transfatty acids.

Guar gum (Cyamopsis tetragonolobus) and glucomannan can be used to reduce body weight and enhance satiety. Psyllium seed husk (Plantago ovata) is used similarly to produce bulking and laxative effects.

6) **Gums and Algal Polysaccharides** - are water soluble gel-forming compounds, and are not foods in essence, but are used as artificial food additives i.e. emulsifiers, thickeners and stabilisers. They have therapeutic

laxative effect. Examples are kraya and gum arabic. Seaweed origin alginic acid, agar and carrageenan are also additives, though agar is used as a laxative, but carrageenan may have adverse effects such as causing ulceration and other intestinal damage, possibly colon cancer, birth defects and hepatomegaly (precise reasons are unclear). Alginate is particularly useful in inhibiting the uptake of heavy metals from the gut, and promoting their excretion, including those exhibiting radioactivity. Galactans also occur in seaweed's. Other NSP's to consider are mannans and dextrans which are used as plasma substitutes in therapy.

Let us now look at the role of fibre, the results of lack of fibre in diet, and the problems that can result from overtake.

1/ Fibre shortens transit time for the passage of material in the gut, especially the large bowel. Thus, dilution and elimination of toxins and carcinogens, bile acids and heavy metals is enhanced. Cholesterol re-absorption is diminished, thereby reducing desoxycholates and steroid metabolism. Thus, fibre can be said to have an anti-atherogenic effect, and an aid to reducing heart conditions, gall bladder disease and cancer of the colon (in addition to intestinal bacterial effect). A larger, softer bulkier stool results, so reducing pressure and straining on evacuation and preventing constipation, diverticulitis, haemorrhoids etc., and probably appendicitis and Crohn's disease.

2/ Dietary fibre increases the transit time in the upper intestinal tract commencing in the mouth, with extra chewing being required. Hence food passes more gradually into the small intestine, pancreatic enzyme activity increases and a more complete digestion takes place, and blood glucose levels rise more slowly and reducing insulin secretion. There appears also to be an increased tissue sensitivity to insulin. The short chain fatty acids produced by the increased dietary fibre seem to enhance liver glucose metabolism. Glucose tolerance is improved and obesity is decreased and prevented; and serum lipid is reduced.

There is a problem with high intake of certain kinds of fibre foods (wheat bran in particular), and this is the presence of phytic acid. Its function in plants is to store minerals such as calcium, phosphorus, magnesium; and dietary phytates can adversely affect the uptake and utilisation of the same calcium, iron, zinc and magnesium. This occurs in unleavened bread i.e. Chapatti and kubz, while in leavened bread the phytase can destroy phytic acid as also may heat. Vitamin C may reduce the phytic acid effect and prevent the mineral absorption deficiencies incurred. Hence, any fibre supplement should not rely on cereal bran (though oat bran has less phytate than the others and more water soluble gels and mucilaginous fibres), but on a mixture of dietary fibres. Thus, any supplementary fibre should be taken away from mealtimes with at least ½ to 1 litre of mineral water.

Though, as previously indicated, specific supplements exist, the best method of supplementation is considered to be whole foods e.g. wholemeal bread, oatmeal products, brown rice, brown pasta, jaggery (brown raw sugar) together with leafy vegetables (lightly cooked, steamed) such as brussel sprouts, cauliflower, mature leguminous seeds, nut and raw vegetables such as watercress. Wheat grass, alfalfa sprouts and chlorella (cracked cell walls) also provide fibre and total nutrition. The important factor is for persons and medical/health practitioners to be aware of the need to increase the daily intake of dietary fibre in its various forms to around the daily recommended norm of 30 grams.

The physicochemical infrastructure of the primary cell wall (see diagram) seems to be important at the molecular level, so providing a matrix which can, in effect be considered as a highly ordered super molecule.

It is known that bile acids in the faeces are strongly adsorbed to the solid components of the stool. The fibrous matter seems to afford protection against the atherogenic effects of dietary fat. Thus, in retrospect, these findings are potentially important because of the possibility that low fibre diets predispose to gallbladder disease, ischaemic heart disease and colon cancer; possibly by diluting and absorbing carcinogens.

Certainly, Diverticular disease of the colon (according to work of Neil S. Painter in Topics in Gastro-Enterology), the aetiology and pathogenesis of such is related to low fibre diet, and processed and refined foods intake.

Various considerations have given rise to the concept that fibre can act as a natural controller of energy balance, so preventing over-nutrition and obesity, and experiments have indicated that fibre induces satiety and limits food intake; and probably high calorie intake. Certainly, recent work indicates that fibre has an insulin-sparing effect, probably due to the slower absorption of glucose. This has implications in the prevention of diabetes and indeed in its treatment, as also in the management of obesity. The concept here revolves round rapid, above the threshold rate, blood glucose level where some of it becomes fat in the liver, under the influence of hyperinsulinism, which increases the synthesis of fatty acids and tri-

Consequences of a high intake dietary fibre

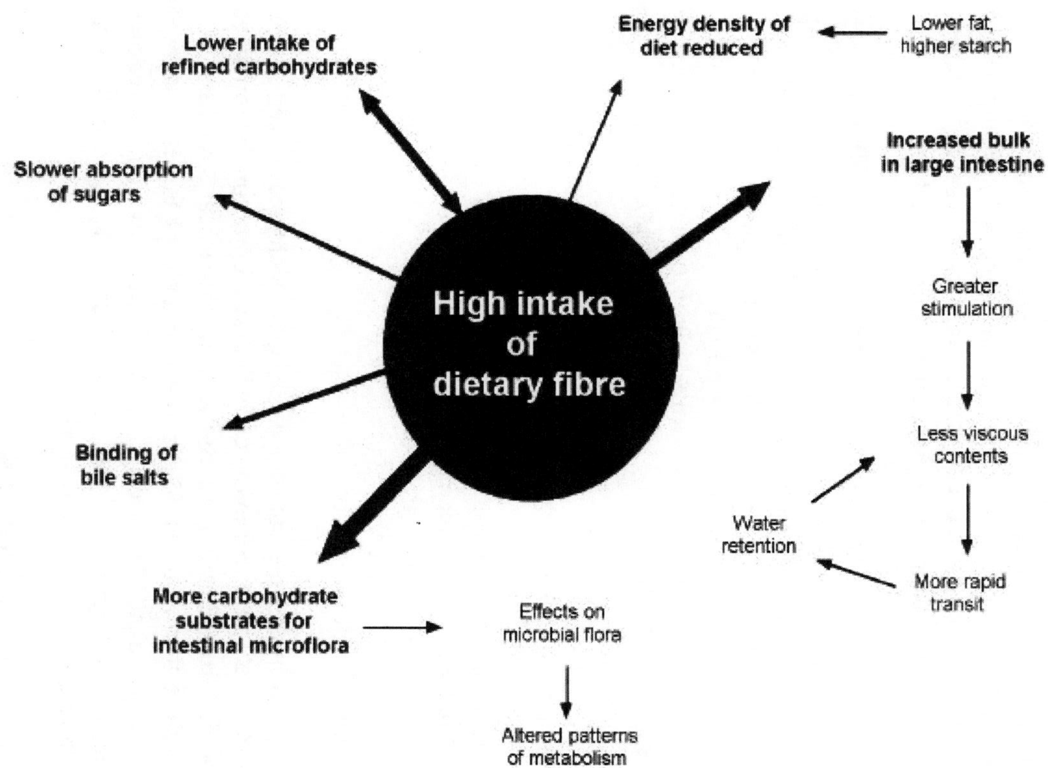

glycerides by adipose tissue/liver, and by increasing the intake of circulating tri-glycerides into adipose tissue by activating lipoprotein lipase.

Gums, mucilage's and pectin's, finally, are high viscosity types of dietary fibre which have marked effects on fat and carbohydrate metabolism, while also decreasing serum cholesterol, and reducing urinary glucose in diabetes, and reducing post-prandial insulin secretion; while also they are used as obesity control agents, especially the galactomannan in guar gum - from the cluster bean. Certainly they play a role in the stability and support of bowel micro flora and in supporting therefore, the mucosal immune system (MIC) in total and possibly in the Immunomodulation factors.

In conclusion two recently discovered forms of NSP on dietary fibre have found favour - such may also have prebiotic action. One, the result of research carried out at the University of Florida, is derived from grapefruit rinds - it is mainly pectin based; contains guar gum, both of which are complexed to soy protein into a powder. This powder is then able to be blended into drinks, soups or mixed with oatmeal (itself high in fibre and possessed of cholesterol lowering properties), sauces etc., soups and casseroles.

Research studies have shown:

1) Cholesterol lowering significantly
2) Improvement in glucose tolerance in diabetes
3) Athero-sclerosis regression
4) Intestinal Flora enhancement
5) Significant weight reduction

The 2nd interesting substance is a glycobiological called Arabinogalactan (AG). AG is a complex carbohydrate, common in tomatoes, but best sourced from certain parts of the North American larch tree. It is available in tablet form, but as AG is water soluble, it is easily incorporated into soups etc. And, because AG doesnt break down until it reaches the large intestine, it doesnt provoke gas or bloating as some prebiotics do. It is therefore suitable for the elderly.

The G.I. effects of AG are 3 fold:

1) It helps to cleanse and detoxify the system by acting as a natural stool softener.

Consequences of low intake of dietary fibre

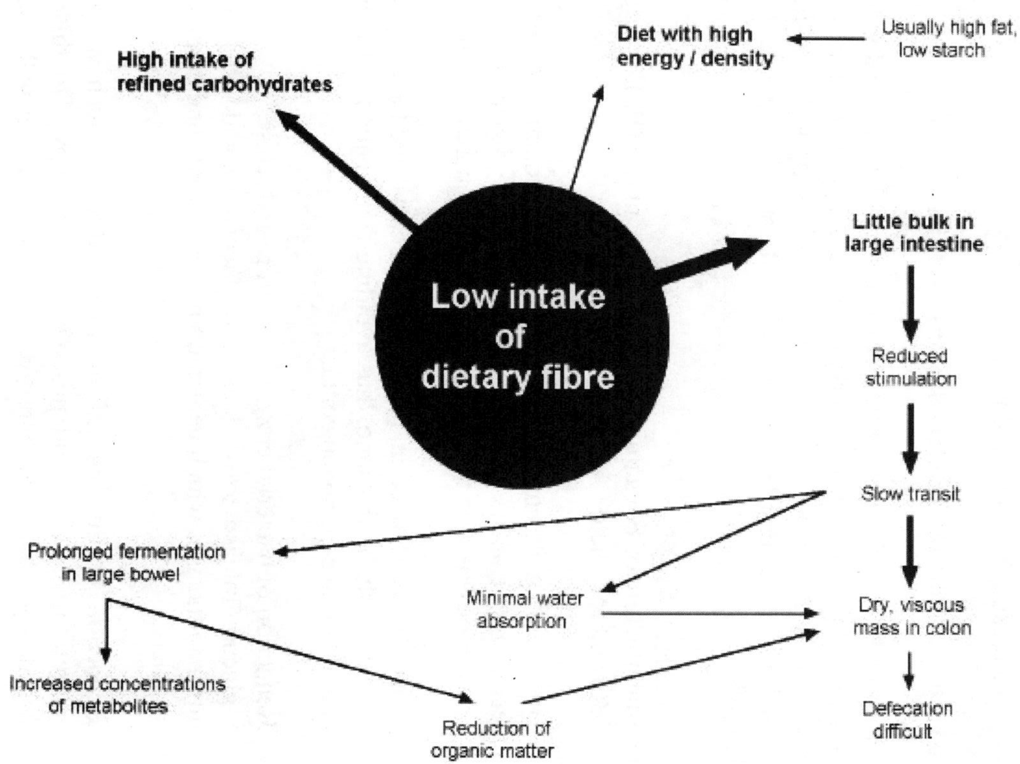

2) It reacts with existing intestinal bacteria to ferment and produce SCFAs and promotes lower (more acid) pH of colon.
3) University of Minnesota (peer reviewed) research indicates that AG increased total micro flora by x 10, after 21 days and decreased pathogenic organisms by 18.5%.

In addition AG seems to keep insulin levels low, decreasing the generation of and absorption of faecal ammonia and as an I.S. booster, by stimulating and by increasing NK cell production.

Part 1.6.1 - Normal Bacterial Flora - Adults

Prior to looking at the individual intestinal floral bacteria individually, it is important to portray a brief overview of their symbiotic function. These are based on conclusions of the expert panel, supported by the EU and founded in November 1995 called LABIP - Lactic Acid Bacterial Industrial Platform.

a) Established Effects:

1) Manufacture of B-vitamins, such as biotin, niacin (B3), pyridoxine (B6) and folic acid.

2) By providing the enzyme lactase, leading to reduction of signs of lactose intolerance, and hence they enhance the digestion of milk based foods, as also thereby calcium absorption and assimilation.

3) Enhance bowel function, especially peristalsis, and hence speed of food through the intestine, thus avoiding constipation, fermentation, and potential carcinogen contact.

4) Reduction of bacterial enzymes i.e. Nitro-reductase, b-glucumomidase, azo-reductase, b-glucosidase and urease, nitrate/ nitrite reductases which generate toxic, genotoxic and carcinogenic products.

5) Reduction of duration of diarrhoeal diseases such as rota virus, enterotoxic E. Coli, and post antibiotic therapy. In this respect a 'pseudo' probiotic Saccharomyces boulardii, a non pathogenic yeast, has been used in many countries, as both a preventative and therapeutic agent for diarrhoea and other gastrointestinal disturbances caused by the administration of antibiotics. S. Boulardii inhibits the growth of a number of microbial pathogens in vivo and in vitro - including Clostridium difficile (see later).

6) Lowering of LDL Cholesterol effects, and thus protecting against cardiovascular damage.

7) Enhancing effects on the Immune System (particularly the humoral element) see later. Alongside this situation the flora plays a role in protecting against the negative effects of radiation (including radiotherapy), chemotherapy and exo and endo toxins (pollutants in particular).

8) Certainly, the flora provides competitive exclusion of intestinal pathogens, as well as providing natural antibiotics as previously mentioned, and hence the flora can be considered per se as providing increased resistance against infections.

9) In various ways the flora provides cancer prevention potential effects.

Prior to considering the establishment of the flora, it is considered convenient to consider each common member of the flora individually.

Much of the detail below is adapted from the original work of Professor Jeremija Lj. Rasic PhD of the Food Research Institute Novi Sad of then Yugoslavia.

MICRO-ORGANISMS USED AS PROBIOTICS

by Dr. Jeremija Lj. Rasic, Ph.D.

1. **Lactobacillus Kefir (Causcasicus)**

A non-resident, i.e. Transient bacteria of the human intestine. Found in kefir grains and drink kefir. Facultative anaerobic (grow in the presence or absence of air) lactobacilli which produce lactic acid, alcohol-ethanol or acetic acid and carbon dioxide from carbohydrates. As with other lactic acid bacteria these transient lactobacilli encourage, because of their formation of lactic acid, etc., a more acid environment in which there is a strong inhibition of less desirable micro-organisms.

2. **Lactobacillus Acidophilus**

A natural inhabitant of the human small and large intestine. Found in the intestine of humans and animals, human mouth and vagina. Facultative anaerobic lactobacilli which produce lactic acid as a main product from carbohydrates. Optimum growth temperature 35 - 38°C.

The major beneficial functions of acido-bacteria are:

a) They enhance and allow digestion of milk sugar (lactose) by producing the enzyme lactase; and generally aid in the digestion of nutrients.

b) They are able by some competitive means e.g. Creation of lactic acid and other inhibitory substances, to suppress undesirable micro-organisms in the intestine.

c) Some strains act to help destroy hostile invading bacteria by producing natural antibiotic substances.

d) Some strains are able to help reduce the level of cholesterol thus lessening the dangers of cardiovascular complications.

e) They are able to lessen the proliferation of hostile yeast's such as Candida albicans/tropicalis.

When the intestinal microflora is disturbed (the lactobacilli can be adversely affected) under the influence of oral antibiotic therapy, or stress conditions, the use of supplemental acidophilus bacteria, in food or concentrated form, can help reverse such negative processes. The regular use of acidophilus bacteria as a supplement or in food is a protective means against an imbalance of the intestinal microflora.

3. **Lactobacillus Bulgaricus**
A transient, i.e. Non-resident of the human intestine, yet important bacteria in human ecology. Together with **Streptococcus thermophilus** constitutes a yoghurt culture which is used in the preparation of yoghurt. Found in yoghurt and cheese. Facultative anaerobic lactobacilli which produce lactic acid as a main product from carbohydrates. Optimum growth temperature 40-43°C. Some strains produce natural antibiotic substances. When eaten or taken supplementally these bacteria can benefit humans by enhancing digestion of milk sugar by producing the enzyme lactase. As with other lactic acid bacteria these transient bacteria encourage, because of their creation of lactic acid, a more acid environment in which there is a strong inhibition of less desirable microorganisms.

4. **Lactobacillus Plantarun**
A transient bacteria of the human intestine. Found in dairy products, sauerkraut, pickled vegetables, silage, cow dung and the human intestine and stools. Facultative anaerobic lactobacilli which produce lactic acid as a main product from carbohydrates. Optimum growth temperature 30-35°C. As with other lactic acid bacteria they encourage, because of their formation of lactic acid, a more acid environment in which there is a strong inhibition of less desirable microorganisms.

5. **Lactobacillus Casei subspecies rhamnosus**
A transient bacteria of the human intestine. Found in milk and cheese, dairy products, cow dung, silage and the human intestine and mouth. Facultative anaerobic lactobacilli which produce lactic acid as a main product from carbohydrates. Optimum growth temperature around 37°C. As reported, these bacteria may be effective in the treatment of certain intestinal conditions; however, more evidence is needed.

6. **Lactobacillus Brevis**
A transient bacteria of the human intestine. Found in milk, kefir, cheese, sauerkraut, silage, cow manure and the intestine and mouth of humans. Facultative anaerobic lactobacilli which produce lactic acid, alcohol (ethanol) or acetic acid and carbon dioxide from carbohydrates. Optimum growth at about 30°C. Some strains produce natural antibiotic substances. Evidence is lacking about the beneficial functions of these bacteria in the intestine; except that as with other lactic acid bacteria they encourage, because of their formation of lactic acid, a more acid environment which is inhibitory to less desirable microorganisms.

7. **Lactobacillus Salivarius**
A natural resident of the human intestine. Found in the mouth and intestinal tract of humans and hamsters, and intestinal tract of chickens. Facultative anaerobic lactobacilli which produce lactic acid as a main product from carbohydrates. Optimum growth at 35-40°C. As with other lactic acid bacteria they encourage, because of their creation of lactic acid, a more acid environment in which less desirable microorganisms is inhibited. More evidence is needed about the beneficial functions of these bacteria in the human intestine.

8. **Lactobacillus Yoghurti (Lactobacillus jugurti)**
Valid name: Lactobacillus helveticus, strains which do not ferment sugar maltose. A transient bacteria of the human intestine. Found in sour milk, cheese (particularly Emmenthal and Gruyere) and cheese starter. Facultative anaerobic lactobacilli which produce lactic acid as a main product from carbohydrates. High acid producers, up to 2% lactic acid. Optimum growth temperature 40-42°C. Evidence is lacking about the possible beneficial functions in the human intestine; except that as with other lactic acid bacteria these bacteria encourage, because of their formation of lactic acid, a more acid environment which is inhibitory to less desirable microorganisms.

9. **Bifidobacterium Bifidus**
A natural inhabitant of the human intestine, but also found in the human vagina. Occur in larger numbers in the large intestine than in the lower part of the small intestine. B. bifidum together with other bifidobacteria species are the predominant organisms in the large intestine of breast-fed infants accounting for about 99% of the microflora. In adolescents and adults, bifidobacteria are a major component of the large intestinal microflora. The levels of bifidobacteria decline with age and also in various conditions of ill-health. They produce acetic and lactic acids, with small amounts of formic acid from fermentable carbohydrates. Anaerobic bacteria with optimum temperature for growth 37-41°C.

The major beneficial functions of bifidobacteria are:

a) The prevention of the colonisation of the intestine by invading pathogenic bacteria or yeast's with which they compete for nutrients and attachment sites.
b) The production of acetic and lactic acids which lower the pH (increase the acidity) of the intestine thus making the region undesirable for other possibly harmful bacteria.

c) The retention of nitrogen and assisting of weight gain in infants.
d) The inhibition of bacteria which can alter nitrates in the intestine (derived from food or water) into potentially harmful nitrites.
e) The production of B vitamins.
f) Assisting in the dietary management of liver conditions.

When the intestinal microflora is disturbed (and consequently bifidobacteria declined) under the influence of oral antibiotic therapy, therapeutic irradiation of the abdomen, reduced gastric acidity, impaired intestinal motility, stresses or some other conditions, the use of supplemental bifidobacteria or in food can restore the intestinal microflora.

10. **Bifidobacteria Infantis**
A natural inhabitant of the intestine of human infant, but also occur in small numbers in the human vagina. Together with other bifidobacteria such as B.bifidum, B.breve they are the predominant bacteria in the large intestine of infants. Anaerobic bacteria which produce acetic and lactic acids and small amounts of formic acid from carbohydrates.

The major beneficial functions are similar to those of B.bifidum.

When the micro flora of infants is disturbed (and the levels of bifidobacteria declined) under the influence of sudden changes in nutrition, use of antibiotics, vaccination, convalescence or sudden weather changes, the use of supplemental bifidobacteria or in food can help in the nutritional restoration of the intestinal micro flora.

11. **Bifidobacterium Longum**
A natural inhabitant of the human intestine. Found in the stools of human infants and adults. Together with bifidobacteria such as B. Bifidum, B. Infantis and B. Breve they are the predominant bacteria in the large intestine of infants. Separate biotype of B. Longum occur in large numbers in the large intestine of adolescents and adults. Anaerobic bacteria which produce acetic and lactic acids with smaller amounts of formic acid from carbohydrates. A wider range of carbohydrates fermented compared with that of B. Bifidum, as:

a) The prevention of colonisation of the intestine by invading pathogens with which they compete for nutrients and attachment sites.
b) The production of organic acids which increase the acidity of the intestine and thereby inhibit undesirable bacteria.
c) The nitrogen retention and assisting of weight gain in infants.

d) The inhibition of bacteria which alter nitrates to potentially harmful carcinogenic nitrites.
e) The production of B vitamins.

If the intestinal micro flora is disturbed (and the levels of bifidobacteria declined) under the influence of using antibiotics, irradiation of the abdomen with gamma or x-rays, reduced gastric acidity, stress conditions, the use of supplemental bifidobacteria or in food can help in the restoration of the micro flora.

12. **Bacillus Subtilis**
Aerobic spore forming bacteria found in the human intestine in very small numbers. Usually occur in a variety of sources. Causative agent of ropy (slimy) bread. They have been implicated in food poisoning, and therefore may be regarded as undesirable bacteria.

13. **Streptococcus Thermophilus (Enterococcus)**
A transient bacteria, i.e. non-resident, bacteria of the human intestine. Together with Lactobacillus bulgaricus constitutes a yoghurt culture which is used in the preparation of yoghurt. Found in yoghurt and cheese, heated and pasteurised milk. Facultative anaerobic streptococci which produce lactic acid as a main product from fermentable carbohydrates. Some strains produce antibiotic-like substances. Optimum growth temperature 40-45°C. As with other lactic acid bacteria these transient bacteria encourage, because of their creation of lactic acid, a more acid environment which is inhibitory to less desirable bacteria. When eaten or taken supplementally these bacteria can benefit humans by enhancing digestion of milk sugar by producing the enzyme lactase. These bacteria are the only streptococci which produce lactase; and they produce it even more than Lactobacillus bulgaricus.

14. **Streptococcus Faecium (Enterococcus)**
A resident bacteria of the human intestine, and occurring in small numbers. Sources: faeces of humans and animals; insects and plants. Usually found in non sterile foods. Facultative anaerobic streptococci, called enterococci which produce lactic acid as a main product from carbohydrates. Used as a starter (in some dairies) for the manufacture of some kinds of cheese. They are resistant to unfavourable environmental conditions, including acidity, temperature, salt, drying, atmospheric oxygen, etc. Scarce scientific evidence about the possibly beneficial functions of these bacteria in the human intestine; especially when compared with acidophilus bacteria and bifidobacteria.

15. **Streptococcus Faecalis (Enterococcus)**
A resident bacteria of the human intestine, and occurring in small numbers. Sources: faeces of humans and animals; insects and plants. Facultative streptococci, called enterococci which produce lactic acid from carbohydrates; some biotypes digest casein and gelatine. They are resistant to unfavourable environmental conditions. They can produce higher than normal levels of amines such as tyramine and histamine in the cheese; and tyramine for example may be involved in the onset of migraine attacks in susceptible persons. Normally, these bacteria are not used as a starter for fermented milk products. There is no firm evidence about the possible beneficial effects of these bacteria for humans.

16. **Streptococcus Lactis (Enterococcus)**
A transient bacteria of the human intestine. Sources: raw milk and milk products, plants and non sterile frozen and dry foods. Facultative anaerobic streptococci which produce lactic acid as a main product from carbohydrates. Used as a starter for the manufacture of cheese, particularly cheddar, and as a component of starter for the manufacture of cottage cheese and cultured buttermilk. Some strains produce antibiotic nisin. The beneficial functions of these transient bacteria in the human intestine are comparatively less than those of acidophilus bacteria and bifidobacteria as well as yoghurt bacteria.

There are some successful probiotic bacteria which have specific reported effects (Salminen et al 1996 as reported in proceedings in symposium "Probiotics in Man and Animal" Berlin 1996. Micro -ecology and Therapy."

1/ **Lactobacillus acidophilus** - LFH and DDS I - balances intestinal flora, immune enhancer, adjuvant, adherent to intestinal cells.

2/ **Lactobacillus acidophilus** NCFB 1748 - lowers faecal enzyme activity, decreased faecal mutagenicity, prevention of radiotherapy related diarrhoea, treatment of constipation.

3/ **Lactobacillus GG** (ATCC 53013) Prevention of antibiotic associated diarrhoea, treatment and prevention of rotavirus diarrhoea, treatment of relapsing Clostridium difficile diarrhoea, Crohn's disease, antagonistic against carcinogenic bacteria, vaccine adjuvant.

4/ **Lactobacillus casei Shirota** (wrongly referred to as immunitas). Prevention of intestinal disturbances, treatment of rotavirus diarrhoea, balancing intestinal bacteria, lowering faecal enzyme activities, positive effects in the treatment of superficial bladder cancer, immune enhancer in early colon cancer, immune enhancer.

5/ **Lactobacillus bulgaricus** - produces natural antibiotic bulgarican - from strain DDS 14 - effective against Bacillus subtilis, E. Coli, Proteus vulgaris, Pseudomonas aeriginosa, Staphylococcus aureus - all showing very strong inhibition of test culture; also Clostridium perfringens, Salmonella enteritidis and typhimurium (hopefully the 'new' pathogenic food poisoning strain, DT104). Shahani Cultured Dairy Products Journal Vol 12 (2) 1977

6/ **S. Enterococcus lactis** produces the natural antibiotic nisin.

Some of the lactobacilli produce hydrogen peroxide (H_2O_2) itself an antibacterial.

Bogdanov observed that Lactobacillus bulgaricus possesses potent anti-tumour activity. This is probably due to 3 glycopeptides which he and his associates discovered at the Research Laboratory in Sofia, Bulgaria.

Furthermore, recent work published in the Japan Journal of Paediatrics (1994) by Sugita and Togawa, using a "Probiotic Drug" i.e. The Lactobacillus preparation "Biolactis Powder" (BLP) confirms much of this earlier work. Also, use of this powder was found to improve the recovery time on infants with rotavirus induced gastro-enteritis; while also producing evidence that mutagenicity is decreased using BLP, including the recurrence of superficial urinary bladder tumours in clinical trials (Eur. Urol. Vol 27. (1995)). The administration was 3 gram/day BLP.

Two studies have recently been carried out on Lactobacillus casei Shirota (LcS); firstly increase in faecal Bifidobacteria was noted, together with significant decreases in both faecal B-gluconidase, and B-glucosidase. Lactobacillus acidophilus seems to have similar actions, plus reducing the level of nitro-reductase and azoreductase (all 4 of these enzymes have been implicated as carcinogens). Certain strains of Lactobacilli have been shown to degrade nitrosamines (carcinogenic agents derived from nitrates and nitrites in food and water).

In 1978, a Russian conference reported the use of Koumiss in the treatment of a number of diseases, including non-specific and chronic lung disease, digestive tract disease, myocardial infarction, chronic cholecystitis and chronic entero-colitis (the Irritable Bowel Syndromes and Malabsorption Syndromes today).

Zimmerman et al in Microbiology and Therapy Vol 26 (1997) reported that probiotic bacteria stimulate the non-specific part of the Immune System - macrophages/monocytes and NK cells. Also, B cells proliferate and produce antibodies in response to probiotic stimulation, and research is continuing to confirm recent evidence of T cell stimulation.

It is important to consider the Intestinal Flora as from the mouth to the anus as there are interrelated effects.

The author is grateful to Dr Barry J. Rathbone, Dept. Of Medicine, St. James University Hospital, Leeds UK, as published in Old Herborn University Seminar monographs No1 1990.

1/ The Mouth - Each millilitre of saliva contains between 10,000 and 1 billion (10^9) micro-organisms, but these are well adjusted to their environment and vary between symbiosis (mutually beneficial) and antibiosis (obligately pathogenic), and are present in varying degrees according to conditions. Primarily are the Streptococcus group i.e. mutans (involved in dental caries), S. Sangus, S. Salivarius, and the Lactobacillus group species i.e. L.Casei, L. Plantarium, L. Acidophilus, L. Fermenti, and L. Brevis (these are often found in the coronal plaque and caries lesions).

It is interesting to note that in China and Japan, it is customary to take some green tea after a meal. Apart from the fluoride effects, i.e. the tea exposes the tooth surface to the anti-plaque effect, and the need for fluoride in tooth structure, the polyphenols in green tea inhibit the growth of S.mutans, and inhibit therefore the S.mutans enzymes which allow the bacteria to form larger areas of plaque. If the root canal has become infected, green tea may help prevent further damage due to the polyphenols as antibacterial agents. Also, green tea helps to overcome gingivitis and prevent its progression to periodontal disease, and equally preventing and overcoming 'bad breath' (Kyushu Univ/Osaka Univ. Japan research). Green tea helps to maintain healthy colonies of beneficial intestinal bacteria in the intestine, and promote growth and provide a less favourable environment for undesirable bacteria - an adjunct prebiotic in fact.

Other important groups of oral bacteria, which are certain to influence the intestinal flora, certainly in the newborn and infancy are the Actino myces and Bifido bacterium species together with the Bacteroids species e.g.

Forsythus, gingivalis and intermedius, together with Clostridium and Campylobacter; and many species of lesser importance; many of which have pathogenic potential.

Exposure of the oral tissues to bacteria during and directly after birth leads to the flora developing, and added to by handling, kissing and eruption of teeth. However, the growth of oral indigenous bacteria is influenced by a vast array of factors: oxygen tension, dietary carbohydrates (vary breast/formula milk fed), bacterial acids, bacterial toxins and a variety of enzymes.

2/ <u>The Stomach</u> - generally the highly acidic nature i.e. pH 4-5 allows only acid resistant lactobacilli and streptococci can survive. However, if acidity becomes less intense i.e. pH 5+ then oral and faecal organisms can be isolated - often pernicious anaemia also occurs. But, importantly Helicobacter pylori becomes established; chronic gastritis occurs, and an associated systemic and a local immune response; with specific antibodies, though insufficient to eliminate the organism.

3/ <u>The Small Intestine</u> - this can be considered a 'zone of transition' between the few bacteria in the stomach, and the heavily populated large intestine; Lactobacilli, Enterococci are found together with a few Bifidobacteria, Bacteroides and yeasts depending on the pH of the internal environment, the degree of peristalsis and mucosal secretion. The extent of pancreatic and bile secretion is possibly important, but primarily the presence of the parasite Giardia, and the fungus Candida may determine flora activity in this area; and the 'fibre' content of the diet.

Important here is the presence or not of Clostridium perfringens bacteria, which produce lecithinase, and also have been connected with the occurrence of collagenosis, especially Rheumatoid Arthritis (RA) (Excerpta Medica Amsterdam 1970). Also included in this Olhagen and Mansson publication are Systemic Lupus Erythematosus (SLE), and psoriatic arthropathy. Parallel studies by D[r] Ebringer, Kings College, London, around 1988 concluded that relative numbers of the Klebsiella bacterial species in the stools bore a direct relationship to exacerbation's of Ankylosing spondylitis (AS), as also RA, SLE, myasthenia gravis, motor neurone disease etc. Lactobacillus acidophilus and L.bulgaricus supplementation, together with a sound diet, prevent Clostridium and Klebsiella acting while therefore preventing exacerbation's etc.; and thereby halting progression. In some cases a degree of recovery has occurred;

especially in B27 and HLA-DR4 tissue-type persons (see Leaky-Gut Syndrome section).

4/ <u>The Large Intestine</u>: Lacto and Bifido-bacteria predominate of the various lactobacilli found to inhabit the colon, sometimes transient unfortunately dependent on diet, is Lactobacillus plantarum and which has a number of positive attributes. It is found, in particular, in fermented vegetables, on raw greens (NOT treated with herbicide/pesticides), fish and in the brine of olives. L.plantarum is essential for the development of a favourable flavour and smell in sauerkraut, and the brine of dill cucumber, and some hard cheese. Part of L.plantarums beneficial activity can be attributed to its very high production of lactic acid, and of the essential amino-acids lysine and methionine. Lysine is well known for certain control of herpes simplex virus conditions and the sulphur containing amino-acids methionine for its free radical scavenging activity and for its effectiveness in eliminating toxic metals from the body.

It is now time to consider how after birth the flora becomes established and the effects of breast/bottle feeding.

It is interesting to note that human breast milk today differs from that of 40 years ago; this is probably due to maternal diet changes, including nutrient defects, together with pollution, including endocrine hormone disrupters. This has affected the intestinal flora in the colons of breast fed infants, today however, the predominant bacteria are B.bifidum and B.longum.
Also, of course, it is well known that significant differences exist between breast and bottle fed (cows milk or formula feeds) babies, high counts of bacteroides, Clostridium and E.coli, whereas, via the colostrum in breast fed babies their is a natural defence via the Bifido bacteria against these pathogenic bacteria; while also the colostrum fed baby has a lower (pH 6-7) acidity, compared with acid pH (around 5.0) in breast fed. The BB factor in human milk is implicated. Klebsiella species are also more frequently present in bottle fed baby's, leading to gastroenteritis as also PCDD and PCDF, together with Dioxins, Furans and also atmospheric pollutants. Obviously, in areas of such risk, to supplement Bifidobacteria is safe and wise.

Before birth, as long as the amniotic membrane remains intact, the normal foetus is sterile until shortly before birth. During passage through the vagina the G.I. Tract receives seeding of many micro-organisms from maternal flora and environment. E.coli is obtained in this way, but may not survive in acid Bifidobacteria predominance but certainly does in formula fed infants, where Bifido levels are lower. Clostridium is acquired, but is more or less destroyed in breast feeding (Graphs from Microbiology of Human Digestive Tract. Old Herborn Seminar No1). The air and hospital personnel, and whether or not recent maternal antibiotics are also relevant. Both groups are rapidly colonised by enterobacteriaceae and Streptococcus species.

However, in formula fed group more bacteroides, Eubacteruim, Peptostreptococcus, Veillomella and Clostridium are significantly higher with risk of diarrhoea etc. Also, there seems to be increased susceptibility to Rota and Echo virus conditions (colostrum etc. seems to confer great immunity) and there are different, and more favourable predominance of the 'good' Bifidos. The E.coli serotypes producing the K1 antigen causing meningitis in neonates seems more likely to take hold.

There are also additional factors involved: (apart from pH)

1/ Oxidation - Reduction Potential.
2/ Volatile Fatty Acids - these are desirable, Bifidos produce copious amounts which reduce E.coli and Streptococcus species. Each able to produce diarrhoea's.
3/ Caesarean Section seems to slow the acquisition of favourable bacteria.
4/ Receptors on the intestinal mucosa are affected in favour of E.coli.
5/ Vitamin K deficiency is in the opposite direction as insufficient E.coli and Bacteroides are around in breast feds to produce.
6/ Toxigenic Clostridium difficile, especially in formula fed seem to flourish, perhaps due to lower pH, or maternal antibiotic recent episodes.

1.6.2 - Normal Bacterial Flora - Baby

As long as the amniotic membrane remains intact, the GI tract is sterile and free of bacterial colonies. During birth, as the foetus passes through the vagina there is considerable 'seeding' with many and varied bacteria from the mother and from the environment. Often, as has been determined with Escherichia Coli (E. Coli), the strains acquired are identical to those of the mother. However, the internal environment of the baby's intestine controls the micro-organisms and strains which survive at this early stage. The prime bacteria initially are lactobacilli, enterococci and other coliforms.

Over the last 20-30 years, there has been determined a trend to change the number and type of bifidobacteria in baby and infant GI tracts, probably due to environment - air, water, food and radioactivity, antibiotics (maternal), pesticides and other toxin pollutants and possibly maternal periods on the contraceptive pill. This has resulted in a paradigm change in infant microflora in respect of micro-ecology, with lowered colonisation of bifidobacteria and higher colonisation of bacteroides and lactobacilli (this is especially so in bottle fed babies); the B. infantis group being particularly in decline.

The significance of this change of balance cannot be underestimated, and may have lifelong implications, and is the subject of present day research; especially in respect of the roles of higher than previous levels of B. bifidum, B. breve, B. longum and B. adolescentis. Such change is being related to changes in the special qualities of human breast milk world-wide; together with increasing use of cow's milk directly or indirectly (which contains more bacteroides clostridium and E.coli - whereas the first human mothers milk or colostrum contains substances antagonistic to these bacteria).

Some of Dr Rasic's comments (his contribution to this volume has been previously acknowledged see 1.6.1) are relevant here. He found steadily increasing levels in infants GI tracts of Klebsiella and pathogenic E.coli (some of which were drug resistant), together with lower levels of acidity in the large intestine, resulting in overgrowth of fungi, yeast's and undesirable bacteria - some potentially pathogenic.

Furthermore, recent studies in Canada/USA have detected toxins such as polychlorinated dibenza-p-dioxin (PCCD) and dibenzofurans (PCDF) in human breast milk. In addition, many other toxins have since been detected, from atmospheric, urban water supplies and living areas such as garden-type pesticides, preservatives and 'leakage' from paper products. These and other man-made chemicals are endocrine disrupters (see Part IV) and pro-carcinogenic compounds - also from water.

All of these 'interference's' with the flora may predispose to viral and bacterial diarrhoea's, as direct effects on the flora itself may equally cause - maybe there is a case developing here for supplementation of B.infantis?!

So, the first 2 weeks post natal are crucial in the development of intestinal bacterial colonisation; and at this time the flora undergoes constant change and is most unstable.

Definitions vary, and the timing of weaning varies culturally, in the UK it is recommended around 3-5 months, meantime breast or bottle feeding

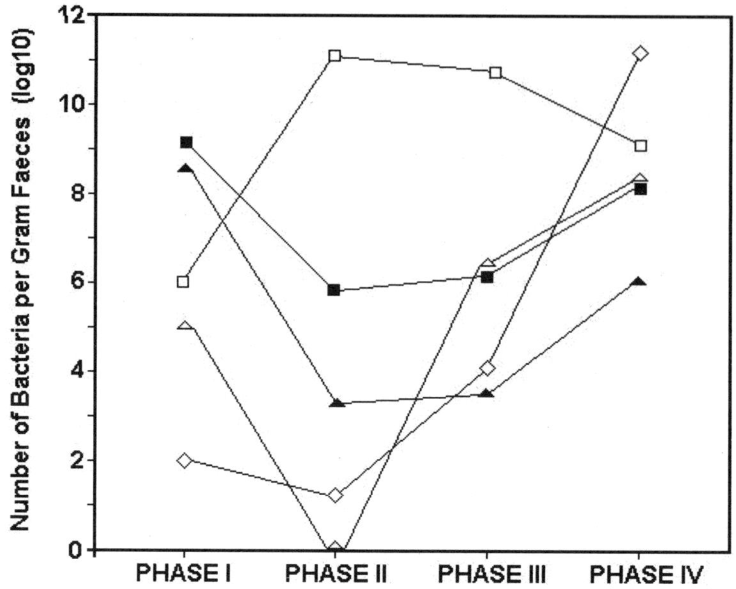

Sequential development of the normal intestinal flora in breast-fed infants

■ : *Enterobacteriaceae;* □ : *Bifidobacterium;* ▲ : *Streptococcus;*
△ : *Clostridium;* ◇ : *other anaerobes*

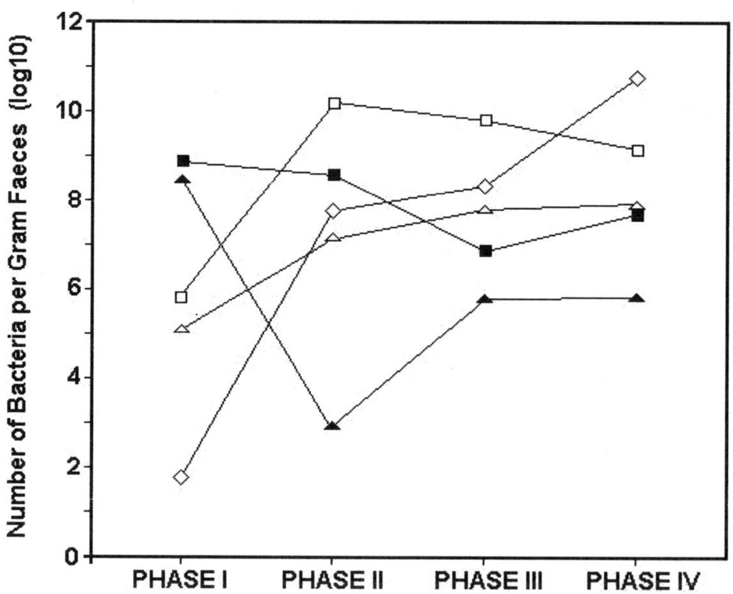

Sequential development of the normal intestinal flora in formula-fed infants

■ : *Enterobacteriaceae;* □ : *Bifidobacterium;* ▲ : *Streptococcus;*
△ : *Clostridium;* ◇ : *other anaerobes*

continues, with perhaps smidgens of formula or cereal food added. The introduction of even these smidgens affects enormously the intestinal ecology, just as the whole system varies (albeit within characteristic patterning) enormously in breast and in formula fed babies and infants (see below). After weaning a baby can be considered an infant.

During weaning and thereafter, the diet influences the flora, indeed such seems to 'trigger' an increase in number of putrefactive bacteroides, generally up to the level of the bifidobacteria, while also lactobacilli also increase. At this weaning stage susceptibility to diarrhoea increases, many of which cases respond to 'probiotics'.

1.6.3 - Normal Bacterial Flora - Infants (post-weaning)

Though some research advocates bifidobacteria for babies, the case is much stronger for infant supplementation of B.infantis (which seems particularly susceptible to toxin disruption) together with L.acidophilus and L.bulgaricus; which together act to inhibit and deactivate pathogens by virtue of the natural antibiotics they produce, and their contribution to favourable acidity levels.

Firstly, in order to appreciate infant GI tract eco-dynamics, the total difference in 'start point' floral content and balance in breast and formula fed babies needs to be considered beyond the Phase IV diagrams in 1.6.2. Generally, in breast fed infants, the 'start point' indicates predominance B.bifidum and B.adolescentis at this stage, while in cows milk based formula fed, B.fragilis predominates, B.adolescentis is lower and 'bacteroides' are noticeable.

As time proceeds the aerobic cross species and anaerobic intestinal flora of formula fed and breast-fed become more and more identical and progress to resembling the adult intestinal flora. There are various consequences and significance's to this state of affairs (some remaining to be elucidated by ongoing research). Certainly, for example, fewer E.coli serogroups are found in the faeces of breast fed infants, than in the faeces of formula fed infants (Braun 1981). It has also been reported that E.coli serotypes containing the KI antigen (known to cause meningitis in neonates) are isolated more often in the faeces of formula fed neonates than breast fed neonates (Orskov & Sorensen 1975) (Braun 1991).

Secondly, research has shown that the 'start point' status quo influences the sequential development of the intestinal flora. In turn, this 'start point' probably affects other factors which influence the sequential development. Some of these factors are outlined below:

1/ Oxidation - Reduction Potential - this is an interesting situation, which in the authors opinion has been insufficiently explored and researched. Little in this sphere has been done since Gritte, Horn and Haenl in 1965, when they purported that the O-R potential of the GI tract immediately after birth is POSITIVE, declines considerably into the negative by weaning and continues to decline to the very "reduced levels characteristic of adults". The "why?" and "whether?" there is any therapeutic implication here, remains in the air.

2/ Volatile Fatty Acids - these are important in the development of neonate intestinal flora - acetic acid predominates - especially in breast fed babies - probably due to Bifidobacteria predominance. Also, proprionic and butyric acids develop later in breast-fed infants, though in formula-fed infants these develop sooner. These acids are inhibitory to a wide variety of bacteria - in some ways perhaps an advantage of formula feeding, but caution in this mode of thinking must prevail - there seems to be little research in this sphere and any secondary effects.

3/ pH - this influences the type of bacteria which can colonise the intestinal mucosa. Again, there is a difference between the pH of breast fed neonates (5.0 - 5.5) and formula-fed neonates (up to 8.5 - very alkaline). Again, little research is evident as to the significance and long term effects of this situation seems to be available.

4/ Babies born by Caesarean Section - seem to show a comparatively low percentage of infants having the presence of B.fragilis - the significance and consequences of this finding seem to be unknown.

There are also geographical differences in neonatal bacterial flora, which is not unsurprising, as also in neonates born prematurely and cared for in incubators, and obviously antibiotic influences take much time for the flora to re-establish normally (including perhaps the antibiotics administered to lactating mothers). Other drugs make changes if transferred into breast milk.

The effects on, and effects of the interaction of the flora, immune system and mucosa cells are considered in 1.3 but must be borne in mind at this stage of baby/infant development, especially the extent of adherence of bacteria to intestinal epithelial cells. The extent of this phenomena must influence the sequential development of neonatal flora. Vitamin K deficiency is an interesting point, such is produced by bacteria in view of its low content in human milk; and maybe due to the reduced numbers of Vitamin K producing bacteria (E.coli, Bacteroides) in breast milk.

Part 1.7 - Control of Flora

The author feels it is important to quote Maarhen P. Hajenberg, Department of Immunology, Erasmus University, The Netherlands. 'Factors responsible for the exclusion of non-indigenous organisms from the intestine and therefore maintenance of floral stability, have not been identified, although several inhibitory mechanisms have been proposed.

They include:

1/ Competition between the flora and non-indigenous organisms for nutrients present in limited quantities.

2/ Elaboration of substances by the flora that inhibit multiplication of non-indigenous organisms e.g. volatile fatty acids in concentrations that can prevent multiplication of S.enteritidis at low pH and oxidation-reduction potential.

3/ Competition between the flora and non-indigenous organisms for attachment sites on the intestinal mucosal cells, and

4/ Establishment of environmental conditions by the flora that adversely affect non-indigenous organisms.

Any one or all may be operative.

It is to be noted that in vivo studies indicate that treatment with streptomycin antibiotic was associated with a decrease in total volatile fatty acids and an accompanying increase in O-R potential and pH producing conditions that favoured the multiplication of S.enteritidis. Similar situations occurred in 'seeding' with Shigella sonnei, S.flexneri and S.dysenteriae. Such indicates that the high concentration of volatile fatty acids, the low (acid) pH and O-R potential are major factors inhibiting multiplication of these species, as also Salmonella and Clostridium difficile."

There are many other controlling factors:

1/ Normal Peristaltic Action - causes a 'nowhere to rest' situation, thereby interfering with replication. Slowing of this action leads to overgrowth.

2/ Stomach Acid Levels - this controls population and also controls yeast levels - (beware use of antacids!) as fewer harmful bacteria are necessary thereby to establish infections.

3/ Interaction of One Type of Bacteria with Another. This state of affairs is variable and hence the pattern of colonisation. Now, the bifidobacteria require an oxygen free environment to thrive, thus a plethora of O_2 dependent bacteria are required to ensure this state and maintain their predominance and hence a healthy patterning. Acidity levels also contribute to this status quo.

4/ Antibiotics undoubtedly 'kill off' and upset the balance and pattern of the intestinal flora, with devastating consequences 'opportunistic bacteria' thrive especially Pseudomembranous enterocolitis, which is the result of proliferation 'grandiosum' of Clostridium difficile. This organism is a toxin producer, and the toxin is a very powerful destroyer of the colonic intestine surface, leading to ulceration, pain and bloody diarrhoea.

Other pathogens, including Staphylococcus aureus, Pseudomonas and Proteus can take over, while OVERWHELMING SUPER (Multiple Resistance) INFECTION can SUPERVENE. The other SUPER INFECTION that can establish itself is CANDIDA, and such has far reaching consequences (see Part II).

5/ Sex Hormones - both natural and artificial (in the form of the contraceptive pill, which in turn seems to act differently in the presence of antibiotics).

6/ Stress - this was considered in 1.4, and this includes radiation effects and infra-sound effects. The question of microwave effects on the flora remains contentious.

And finally,

7/ Dietary effects. This revolves around 2 key factors:

a) Fibre - non-starch polysaccharides (NSP) intake. This is considered in depth in 1.5.

b) Animal Protein / Fat Intake - the high protein diet (mainly meat and hence saturated animal fat) so characteristic of industrialised, so-called Western Society, creates problems in respect of the flora. Firstly, there is an increase in colonic bacteria, which produce the enzyme fadehydroxylase compared with more vegetarian orientated diets. The significance of this seems to be related to the fact that persons suffering from colon cancers have also such high levels. Secondly, in heavy meat eaters the faeces contain high levels of coprostanol and copro-stanone. These are end-products of cholesterol breakdown and are known to be potential carcinogenic agents. These substances and the excess enzyme fa-dehydroxylase are indicators of dietary determinants modifying the intestinal flora, and the need to degrade cholesterol, and breaking down bile acids to secondary bile acids. Researchers have also concluded from studies of variations in intestinal bacterial flora that 'Long term vegetarian diets decrease the metabolic activity of the faecal microflora (in contradistinction to above) and thereby tending to reduce the incidence of colon cancer'.

8/ <u>Natural Antibiotic Action.</u> The intestinal flora possess natural antibacterial, anti-viral and anti-fungal properties, together with the ability to produce hydrogen peroxide (H_2O_2), and various acids. The exact point in time, when such are developed, and whether any exact controlling factors operate is undetermined, but obviously supplementation must enhance the situation amongst other positive effects.

A summary is outlined below:

1/ Bifidobacteria sp produce	Bifidin
2/ Lactobacillus acidophilus produce	Acidolin
(DDS 1)	Acidophillin
	Lactobacillin
	Lactocidin
3/ Lactobacillus bulgaricus (DDS 14)	Bulgarican
4/ Lactobacillus plantarum	Lactolin
5/ Streptococcus lactis	Nisin

Acidophillin has been researched to inhibit the following:

a) Salmonella typhosa (typhi)
b) Shigella species
c) Staphylococcus aureus
d) Pseudomonas fluorescens and the more common P.aeruginosa
e) Klebsiella pneumoniae
f) Vibrio comma, and positive effects on V.parahaemolyticus but not just the antibiotic properties, but also due to the lactic acid and H_2O_2 production.

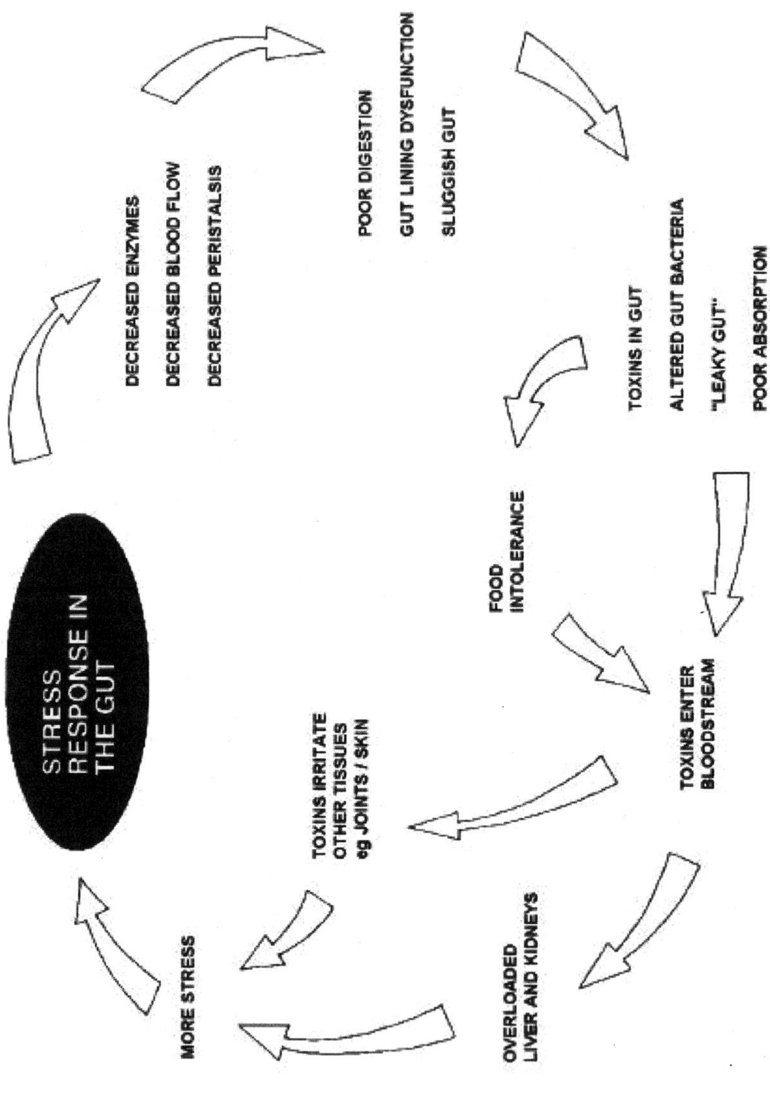
STRESS RESPONSE IN THE GUT
DECREASED ENZYMES
DECREASED BLOOD FLOW
DECREASED PERISTALSIS
POOR DIGESTION
GUT LINING DYSFUNCTION
SLUGGISH GUT
TOXINS IN GUT
ALTERED GUT BACTERIA
"LEAKY GUT"
POOR ABSORPTION
FOOD INTOLERANCE
TOXINS ENTER BLOODSTREAM
TOXINS IRRITATE OTHER TISSUES eg JOINTS / SKIN
OVERLOADED LIVER AND KIDNEYS
MORE STRESS

Positive effects are noted in all kinds of food poisoning especially in infants and in situations of 'travellers diarrhoea' as well as various viral diarrhoea's. Candida, as will be seen later, is very much responsive to various flora as above; details will appear later in this book, as also positive effects in terms of other yeast's, fungal overloads.

Part 1.8 Anti-Mutagenic Effects of Intestinal Flora

Doll & Peto in 1981 produced epidemiological studies indicating that around 1/3 of all human cancers were related to diet; and such studies were followed up by published studies that the presence of natural mutagens, anti-mutagens and cancer modulating compounds are present in human food.

Sigimura 1982 concluded that there is a close relationship concerning certain carcinogens acting as mutating agents, and that these originated from food and environment.

Lactic Acid bacteria and their fermented food products probably render therapeutic benefits, including anti-mutagenic and anti-carcinogenic activity; and it is well known that carcinogenesis is initiated by mutation. Some of the species and strains have been shown to exhibit anti-mutagenic activities against organic nitrogen mutagens.

Part 1.9 - Anti-Tumour Effects of Lactic Acid Bacteria

This is a complex subject, most out of the scope of this book, for it involves injection of lactic acid bacteria either intraperitoneally, intravenously, sub-cutaneously and intratumourally, together with oral intake.

The results of such therapeutics have been researched in depth, but the exact mechanisms are still only partly known. However, favourable effects using oral administration have been demonstrated via studies on M cells or macrophages in the Peyer's patches. Thus, they, having ingested the lactic acid bacteria by phagocytosis they initiate intestinal local immune responses by causing trans-epithelial migration of bacterial antigens from the lumen into the lymphoid tissues. Thus, such action potentiates the host immune system and induces anti-tumour activity.

Part II : The Intestine in Disease

2.1 Dysbiosis - Nature & Significance

The term dysbiosis is used to describe a disturbance from the bio-individualistic optimal state norm of his/her intestinal micro-ecology. Thus intestinal dysbiosis means unbalanced intestinal bacterial flora, which state indeed may be the link between food and lifestyle in its impact on health and disease. These intestinal micro-organisms influence body functions, biochemically and immunologically, hence it is important to treat the microflora in an enlightened probiotic direction.

These probiotics, often some sort of lactic acid producing cultures, are able, together with the host's own flora, to deal with disturbances due to inadequate food, stress and strain - environmental toxins and different medical drugs such as antibiotics, contraceptives, painkillers etc. The intestinal flora influence the immune system and regulate the body's ability to cleanse itself of waste products i.e. detoxification. A harmonised and balanced flora will contribute to a better absorption of nutrients i.e. minerals, trace elements, vitamins and amino acids.

Published research has listed Dysbiosis as a contributing cause in rheumatoid arthritis, autoimmune disease (recently to include Ankylosing Spondylitis - Dr A.Ebrunger, Kings College Hospital, London), where Klebsiella species are implicated, B12 deficiency, chronic fatigue, cystic acne, the early stages of colon and breast cancer, eczema, food allergy/sensitivity, inflammatory bowel disease and IBS, multiple scleriosis, psoriasis, Sjogren's syndrome and steatorrhea.

2.1.2 Suggested signs and symptoms for dysbiosis include allergies, food cravings, overweight, mood swings, hay fever, dry eyes, heartburn, headaches, chronic fatigue, low blood sugar/tiredness, high blood pressure, diarrhoea, constipation, depression, poor memory, more than normal flu and colds, puffy eyes, joint pain, easy bruising, swellings oedema (hives), hyperactivity, difficulty in sleeping, fibromyalgia, muscle soreness, asthma etc.

2.1.3 Candida albicans, Candida tropicalis, Candida cruzei are often found in small (symbiotic) numbers in the Gastrointestinal tract and vagina. It is an opportunistic fungal pathogen which flourishes in carbohydrate-rich environments and other conditions where it can proliferate.

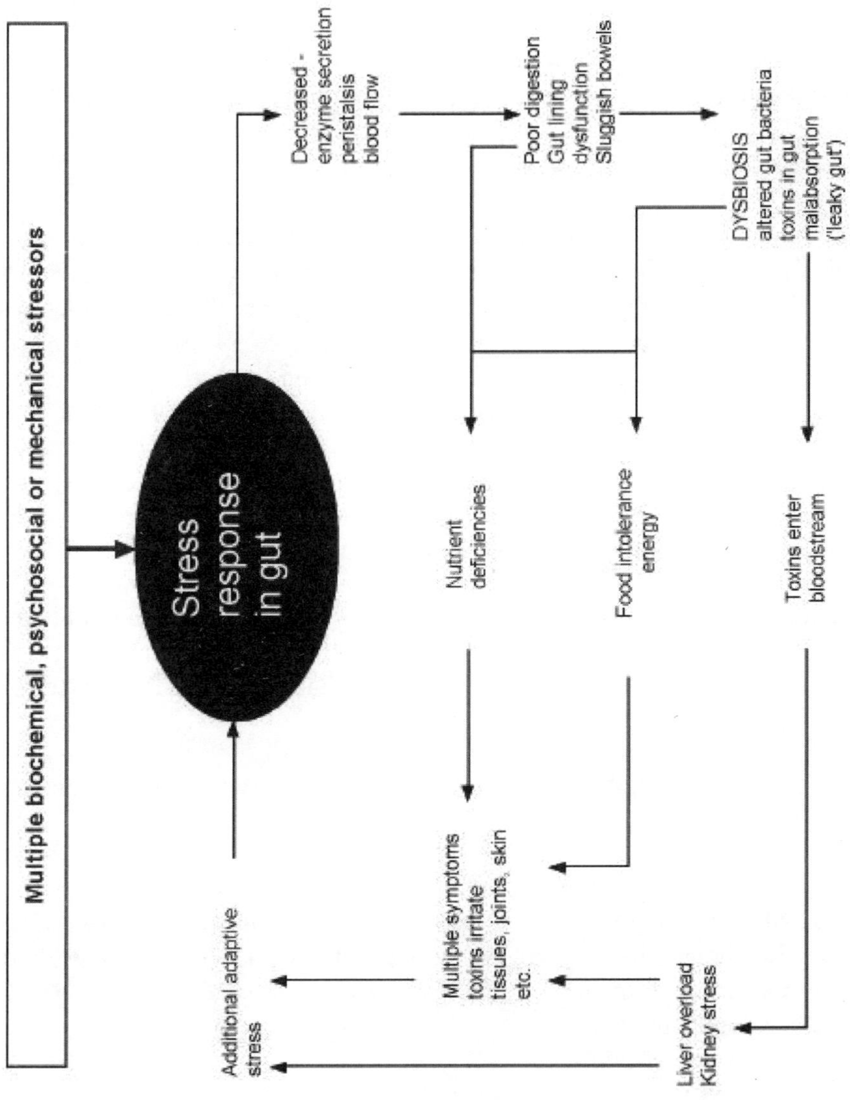

Multiple biochemical, psychosocial or mechanical stressors
Stress response in gut
Decreased - enzyme secretion peristalsis blood flow
Poor digestion Gut lining dysfunction Sluggish bowels
DYSBIOSIS altered gut bacteria toxins in gut malabsorption ('leaky gut')
Nutrient deficiencies
Food intolerance energy
Toxins enter bloodstream
Multiple symptoms toxins irritate tissues, joints, skin etc.
Liver overload Kidney stress
Additional adaptive stress

When Candida proliferates in the intestines, it changes its form from yeast-like to fungal. In its fungal form it produces very long, root-like structures that penetrate the mucous lining of the Gastrointestinal tract wall. As a result dietary proteins, which are incompletely digested, may travel through the blood stream (can often be seen on dark phase microscopy) and attack the immune system, as the penetration breaks the boundary between the Gastrointestinal tract and the bloodstream.

The above causes the immune system to produce large amounts of antibodies, which in turn result in various types of allergies i.e. 'cerebral allergy' with resulting depression, mood swings, and changes in memory, learning ability and behaviour. Certain elements of the Pre-menstrual Syndrome i.e. cravings for sweet foods, cramps, pains, lack of sexual libido, lack of co-ordination and balance, nervous irritability and ear sensitivity may be related to Candida proliferation. Candida itself may get into the bloodstream and can be so seen and transported and exerting systemic effects such a joint pain, chest pain, skin and nail problems and recurrent vaginitis (often in cases on the contraceptive pill).

Candida acts synergistically and amplifies virulence of other pathogenic organisms, and functions as a catalyst in this respect. Equally certain viruses, e.g. cytomegalo virus, can lower resistance to Candida, coxsachiae viruses are similar in effect.

Causes of Intestinal Microflora Imbalances Which Can Lead to Candidiasis

- Antibiotic therapy - maybe 'low key' antibiotics in food
- Steroids - maybe 'low key' steroids in food and supplements
- Hormonal changes caused by oral contraceptives, menopause, post partum adjustments - equally xenobiotic oestrogen's
- Malnutrition
- Gastric operations
- Disturbances of gastric function
- Disorders of intestinal motility
- X-ray irradiation of the abdomen - equally perhaps ultrasound and low frequency noise, loud noise
- Gastric achlorhydria resulting from ageing, or associated with pernicious anaemia
- Stagnation of the intestinal contents due to blind loops
- Disorders impairing intestinal motility, i.e. diverticulosis of the small intestine, regional enteritis

- Gastro-colic and entero-colic fistulae
- Liver cirrhosis
- Disorders of immunological system, e.g. hypogammaglobulinemia
- Stress - psychological, major temperature changes, bright lights etc.

N.B. Gerald Guest - FDA Veterinary Medical Centre

"When you feed antibiotics to animals (as also hormones), you do create populations of organisms that are drug resistant."

- the antibiotics are creating pathogens that cannot be easily controlled by those same antibiotics.

2.1.4 In order to understand shifts in balance and the effects thereof, it is useful to have a comparative diagram. Undoubtedly, today, Candida is developing into epidemic proportions. It is important to realise that lifestyles today are often conducive to forming degenerative intestinal bacteria, rather than a flora which supports the healthy functioning of the body. It is particularly important for a state of health that the balance between the 2 predominant groups of bacteria, the Bifido bacteria and the bacteroides bacteria, is maintained. There is a general tendency for the Bifidobacteria to decline during senescence.

On the next page is a generalised scheme of the human gut microbiota composition. The different bacterial groups are divided on the basis of whether they exert properties which are potentially damaging or health-promoting for the host. The central vertical line gives approximate numbers in faeces

Conjugation and deconjugation

One of the methods the liver uses is to neutralise toxins by conjugating them with glucoronic acid, thereby creating glucuronides. This process is called conjugation. When these are excreted from the gallbladder out into the intestine, certain bacteria's improve their ability to digest these conjugates. This is called deconjugation. The toxins are reabsorbed into the blood. The result is retoxification. Some of the enzymes that deconjugate and retoxify toxic waste products are betaglucuronidase, azoreductase and nitroreductase. The outcome of their action is an increases accumulation of toxic metabolites. By probiosis this will be reduced. Glycosides from different green plants such as rutin may be converted by the action of Streptococcus faecium to quercetin. This

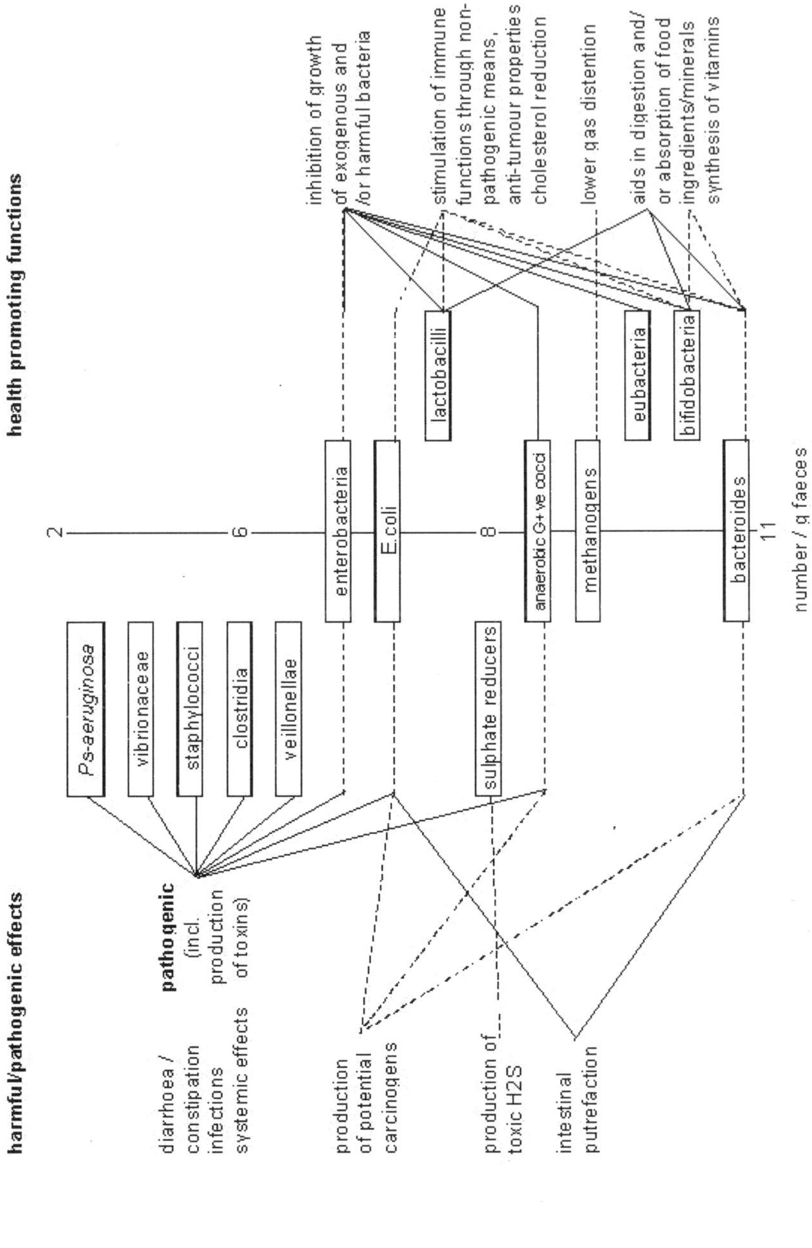

Modified from Gibson & Roberfroid.

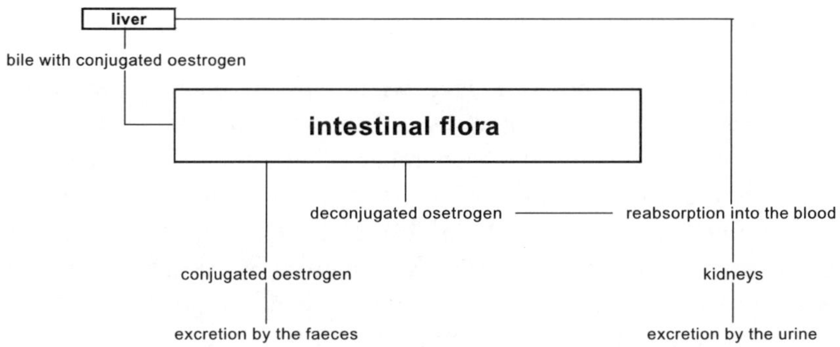

The relationship of the intestinal bacteria and oestrogen and its reabsorption and excretion

molecule is mutagenous. It will cause injuries on the body cell's genetic code. This can develop to malignant conditions i.e. cancer. Streptococcus faecalis is responsible for another sort of retoxification. It converts the amino acid tyrosine to tyrosamine. An increased amount of tyrosamine is thought to trigger attacks of migraine. In a later phase this amine is converted to phenol which is mutagenous.

2.1.6 Oestrogen

Bile acids, cholesterol and a variety of sex hormones are exposed by the same mechanisms i.e. conjugation and deconjugation. They are excreted by the bile into the intestine. Further down in the intestinal channel they are reabsorbed. A certain amount is lost in the faeces. A loss of volatile bile acids and, to a certain degree, cholesterol are lost in the same manner which could be favourable. It is not desirable for the sex hormones to be lost in the faeces. Both female and male hormones can be lost in this manner. This happens when there is intestinal dysbiosis. A reduced concentration of oestrogen can cause bleeding disturbances, increased sensitivity to genital infections i.e. vaginitis and in the bladder i.e. cystitis, impaired fertility and osteoporosis with pain syndrome. You may experience similar mechanisms when taking contraceptives and antibiotics at the same time.

2.2 Dysbiosis - Causes

2.2.1 How does dysbiosis develop?

There are many factors that influence what type of bacteria or micro-organisms there will grow or colonise in the gastrointestinal channel. In the mouth there are already quite a number of bacteria. Many of them come from the intake of food. In the ventricle the amount will be reduced. In the small intestine the numbers of bacterial cells, increase from the beginning towards the end i.e. E10-11/g content. Stress, food, medical drugs, environmental toxic loading and climate are all factors that stimulate or inhibit different types of micro-organisms. A poorly balanced diet will create a dysbiosis.

Different life situations with psychic stress or disharmony are also very influential in creating a dysbiosis. A great number of medical drugs inhibit the beneficial flora from acting normally. Environmental toxins can also provoke an intestinal dysbiosis. Food supplements taken inadequately will disturb the important balance. It should be noted that the climate supports a variety of different bacterial cultures. This is often experienced when travelling i.e. tourist diarrhoea.

2.2.2 Bifidobacterias and bacteroides

What bacteria are there in the stomach and the intestine?

When fasting you only find small quantities in the stomach. Together with the intake of food the amount of bacteria will increase to E5 cfu/ml liquid. There often are streptococci, bifidobacteria, enterobacteria and bacteroides some of them emanating from the mouth and the food itself. These will be reduced when the stomach starts producing acid and the pH is reduced. Further down in the small intestine the number of cells increase again; E5-7 cfu/ml content.

In the colon the numbers increase dramatically. The two dominating types of cultures are bacteroides and bifidobacteria. There are about E10-11 cfu/g faeces. The weight is 0,5-1 kg! The total amount is E14. This is related to the total amount of human body cells that is E13. This implies that there are 10 fold more micro-organisms than body cells! This is of importance especially when referring to the immune system. The Peyer's patches in the small intestine play the most important role in the control and balance of the immune system and it's relation to the microflora.

There is a microeco-intesto-immuno-endocrino-neuro -psycho linkage. This explains many of the syndromes described, where you find both physical and psychiatric disorders closely related to each other.

2.2.3 Fermentation and putrefaction

Simplified you could separate the Bifidobacteria as the good ones and the bacteroides as the evil ones. Bifidobacterias split the food by fermentation. Lactic acid, acetic acid and butyric acid are produced. These will create a more acid environment in the intestine. The bacteroides will digest the food by putrefaction. It will then produce nitrogen waste products. These are harmful for the human body and they will be absorbed in the intestine reaching all the different body tissues. Streptococci, enterococci, enterobacteria i.e. colibacteria are found in minor quantities. In adolescents the quantity of bifidobacteria is lower.

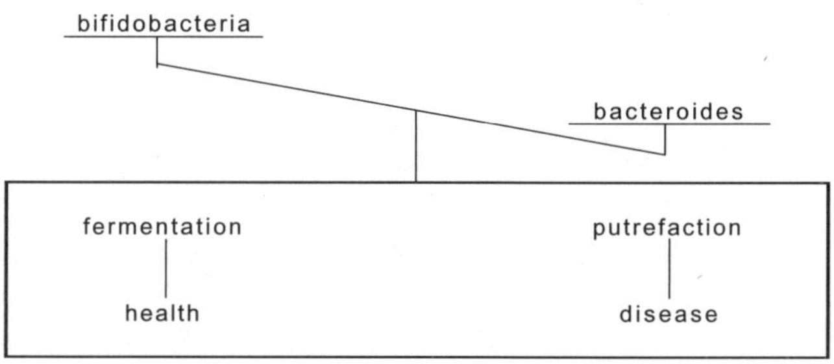

Bifidobacteria and bacteroides live in an ecological balance

2.2.4 What sort of diet promotes a healthy flora?

Food rich in complex carbohydrates with a low glycaemic index. These are broken down relatively slowly and will provide you with a steady blood sugar level. Vegetables of different types, rice and pasta are adequate roughage. A high intake of protein and animal saturated fatty acids stimulate the activity of bacteroides towards putrefaction. In western society we strain our bodies with the intake of too much protein and saturated fatty acids. The WHO standard protein requirement is approximately 0,8 g/day/kg body weight. An intake of high amounts of fibre will improve the motility of the intestine. This promotes the bifidobacteria. A vegetarian diet contains many different food fibres such as cellulose, hemicellulose and pectin. An intake of fibre should always be followed by intake of water. The term 'throw water' is adequate. It indicates enough hydration.

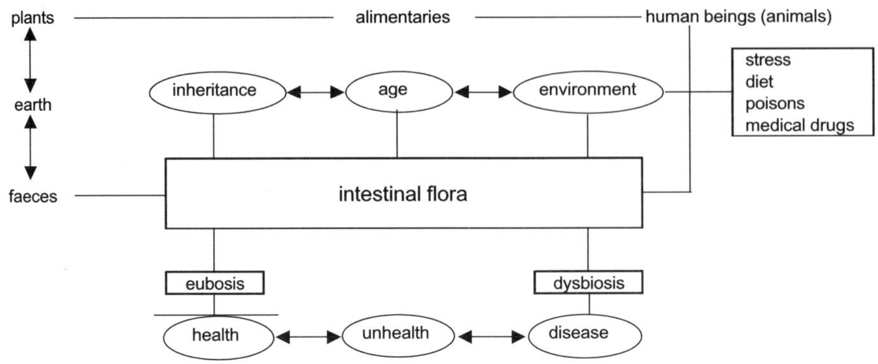

Intestinal dysbiosis and its relation to diseases and the ecological system (Cedgard / Kirkman).

2.2.5 Eubiosis and Probiosis

What are probiotics?

Lactic acid bacterial cultures, so called probiotics, stimulate colonisation of the so called human autochotonous flora in a beneficial direction. Probios means for life. A condition without any dysbiosis is called eubiosis. It is more likely to be an utopia. Reducing the degree of dysbiosis is called probiosis. That is why the cultures are called probiotics. As a therapist you would, of course, advise your patient to optimise all the factors mentioned above. A well balanced diet and life pattern is the best insurance for being healthy. In most cases probiotics could be an important, if not crucial, complement.

2.3 Dysbiosis - Effects

2.3.1 Dysbiosis will often show as functional disturbances in the stomach or the intestine. Symptoms such as dyspepsia, constipation or loose stools are conditions that will later develop into gastritis and chronic inflammation in the intestine. Ulcers in the stomach/duodenum and intestine could result if the dysbiosis is not properly regulated. Gall bladder problems are often related to intestinal dysbiosis.

Dysbiosis is most often seen in relation to dysfunction of the immune system i.e. food intolerance, atopies and allergies i.e. eczema and urticaria are of similar origin. Chronic inflammatory disease i.e. arthritis are also developed in the context of dysbiosis. Certain types of migraine, where food and diet are significant in the situation, could also be a symptom (effect) of intestinal dysbiosis.

2.3.2 In dysbiosis, organisms of low intrinsic virulence, including bacteria, yeast's and protozoa, induce disease by altering the nutrition or immune responses of their host. Published research has implicated intestinal dysbiosis as a cause of Vitamin B12 deficiency, steatorrhea, irritable bowel syndrome, inflammatory bowel disease, autoimmune arthropathies, the genesis of colon and breast cancer, psoriasis, eczema, cystic acne and chronic fatigue.

The mechanisms for these disorders are varied:

Bacteroides cause B12 deficiency by uncoupling the B12-Intrinsic factor complex.
Klebsiella and Proteus are thought to precipitate ankylosing spondylitis and rheumatoid arthritis in genetically susceptible individuals through mimicry of human HLA antigens.
Protozoan infestation can cause arthritis by circulating immune complexes.
Aerobic bacteria may cause irritable bowel syndrome by increasing intestinal prostaglandin synthesis.
Candida albicans causes bowel inflammation through Type 1 hypersensitivity.
Colon carcinogenesis is enhanced by alterations in gut fermentation patterns and bacterial bile salt metabolism.
Altered oestrogen metabolism by gut flora may account for dietary effects on mammary carcinoma.
Activation of the alternative pathway of complement by bacterial endotoxin or yeast zymosan as a result of increased intestinal permeability may underlie the pathophysiology of Crohn's disease, psoriasis and cystic acne.
Amoebic lectins can induce HIV replication in vitro.
Enteroviral antigenemia is a feature of the chronic fatigue immune dysfunction syndrome. Prolonged enteroviral replication results from local immune suppression due to intestinal dysbiosis.

The bowel flora must be normalised for normal immunity in the body. Overgrowth and predominance of organisms are caused by antibiotic usage, histamine antagonists, decreased stomach acid production, birth control pills and poor diet. Any history of bowel problems should cause you to investigate the patient for parasites, protozoans, yeast or bacterial overgrowth. Many clinical syndromes attributable may be caused by any of the above organisms. The use of grape seed extract, garlic, berberine, echinacea, caprylic acid, iodine, Chinese herbs, bowel nosodes, probiotic seeding and dietary restriction for food allergies are more successful than regular chemotherapeutics in rebalancing the flora.

2.3.3 How will dysbiosis be inhibited?

Through the stimulation of beneficial bacteria in the intestine, the degree of dysbiosis will be reduced optimising the food intake and avoiding detrimental stress. Mental and physical welfare can be disrupted by harmful medical drugs, environmental toxins and micro-organisms. There are not many of us that can live in total harmony. This would be an utopia. To be successful in this, you must learn what is beneficial and what is harmful for the intestinal flora in general and in each case.

2.4 Dysbiosis - Investigative Procedures

2.4.1 Clinical Investigation : (best in partnership with physician)

A) History, Signs, Symptoms

A total, holistic and lifestyle history should be taken; including any courses of antibiotics, steroids and any other drug regimes - what they were taken for and how long they were taken.

Specific areas of need to know:

1) Migraine or migraine-type headaches
2) Insomnia, dizziness
3) Respiratory assessment, including hay fever, asthma, recurrent infections (especially ear associated with RA affects)
4) Cardiovascular conditions (including, in some cases, ECG assessment)
5) Gastrointestinal - detailed
6) Skin / muscles / joints
7) Emotions / mind functioning / energy / activity status

B) Clinical Investigations : Laboratory

1) Parasitology and comprehensive digestive stool analysis - often repeated tests are required, including "Candiscan"
2) Full blood test, including liver function, antibody assay (for Ig group) and dark-phase (field) blood microscopy. Allergy (food) sensitivities
3) Intestinal permeability test (mannitol/lactulose) - this is a urine test
4) Breath test - seeking methane, hydrogen from gut putrefaction. Candida
5) Saliva test - seeking stress hormones etc.
6) Food and environmental sensitivity testing
    a) Elimination / provocation testing
    b) Allergy assay
7) Nutritional assay - especially antioxidant status

All of these tests are expensive and need to be undertaken at specialist laboratories by experienced technicians. Usually only a few are necessary: the history, signs and symptoms will be 'Key indicators' and the laboratories usually provide 'interpreted' results. "Before" and "After" probiotic therapy tests may be required. Some practitioners utilise EAV (Voll) or Motoyama Testing Protocols, and EWSA testing.

2.6 Dysbiosis

(CFIDS) - Chronic Fatigue Immunodeficiency Syndrome
(PVFS) - Post-Viral Fatigue Syndrome
(ME) - Myalgic Encephalomyelitis

Chronic Fatigue Syndrome is now recognised by the World Health Organisation as a debilitating and distressing condition. It is multifactorial in origin and presents as a complex symptomatology, as also it has many variant terminologies and criteria as a clinical entity.

These criteria are also complex:

1) Holmes 1988
2) Oxford
3) CDC
4) Australia

It is outside the scope of this book to discuss these. Certain 'key' features are evident in each of the criteria:

1) Environment - intolerance of toxins
2) Allergic - with frequent infections
3) Iatrogenic - multiple courses of antibiotics, steroids, NSAID's, antihistamine drugs
4) Muscular and joint connective tissue, aches and pains
5) Bowel symptoms - dysbiosis, Candidiasis
6) Autonomic Nervous System hyperactivity and PNEI disturbances
7) Disturbance of Hypothalmic-Pituitary-Adrenal-Thymic Axis
8) Viral, metabolic, immunological factors past or present
9) Cognitive dysfunction

There is insufficient space in this book to go into details, but the key immunological indicator is reduction in Natural Killer Cell function, which relates to previous viral infection or stressor related re-activation of viruses dormant.

A plethora of viruses have been implicated:
1/ Herpes Virus I, II, VI, ? VIII (VI may be reactivation)

2/ Enteroviruses
3/ Retroviruses
4/ Epstein-Barr virus (again may be reactivation)
5/ Coxsackie B virus group

Antibodies have been detected and viral RNA have been found in muscles both in CFS and other conditions. Various authorities include fibrositis and fibromyalgia in CFS. Environmental stressors and toxins are implicated, especially many herbicides, pesticides, additives, preservatives, organo-phosphates, organo-chlorines have been specifically singled out as primary or secondary 'triggers'.

Candida is a variant but, invariably, present to some extent as also Dysbiosis, with associated 'toxic overload'.

The treatment protocol needs must be holistic - briefly:

1/ Candida exclusion management
Dysbiosis management see later sections
2/ Environmental management, including food allergies
3/ Detoxification - connective tissue, GI tract, liver
4/ Stimulate oxidative metabolism and establish optimum nutrition

ref : The Clinical & Scientific Basis of ME/CFS, Nightingale Foundation, 1992.

2.6 Leaky Gut Syndrome
(acknowledgements a) Alta Smit - see below, b) Leaky Gut Syndrome. Lipski - Keats, 1998)

2.6.1 Our modern lifestyle produces interference with the normal functioning of the intestinal gut flora. Infections, drugs, certain foods and psychological/technological environmental stress can cause the paracellular pathway to become more permeable or leaky - this resulting in the so-called leaky gut syndrome i.e. increased antigen uptake in the intestinal mucosa.

According to Alta Smit in Bio-Medical Therapy Vol. XVII No.3 1999 'These antigens are transported via the transcellular route, during which neuro-endocrine and immune mediators are activated. Under certain pathological conditions the tight functions between epithelial cells become 'leaky', thus facilitating increased antigen uptake.

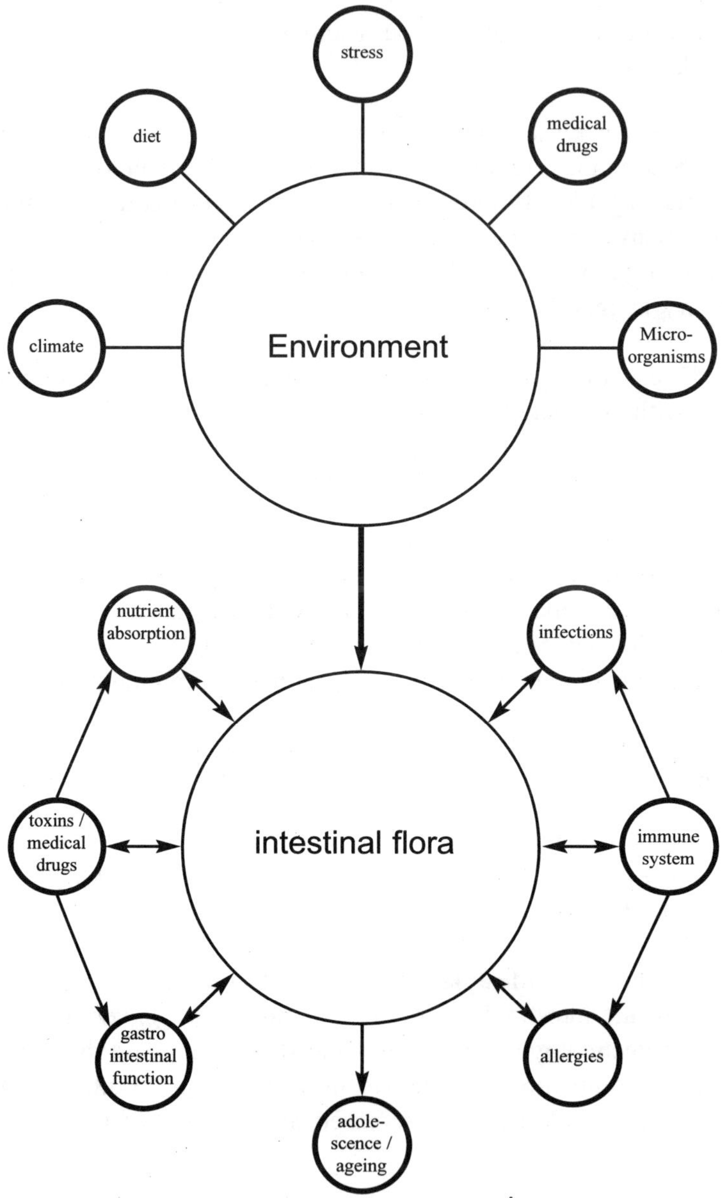
stress
diet
medical drugs
climate
Environment
Micro-organisms
nutrient absorption
infections
toxins / medical drugs
intestinal flora
immune system
gastro intestinal function
allergies
adole-scence / ageing

This results in 4 vicious cycles:

A) allergy and inflammation
B) malnutrition - impaired nutrient absorption
C) bacterial dysbiosis
D) hepatic stress - toxin accumulation

These cycles play a role in the pathogenesis of disease or may contribute to their symptoms.

The gut mucosa can be considered one of the sensory organs. The contents of the gut are from outside the body and it is up to the gastrointestinal mucosa (and its adjacent microflora) to recognise the multitude of substances as either noxious or useful to the body. Thus, the gut needs to act as both barrier and facilitator. The barrier function of the gut is a perfect example of psycho-neuro-endocrine-immunology in action (PNEI).

The extrinsic barrier is made up of the mucus layer and Secretory IgA as well as normal gut flora, which prevent toxins from having direct contact with the epithelial surface. The active barrier is more important and comprises the mucosal epithelium, ion secretion into the lumen, the intraepithelial lymphocytes and the immune system (GALT) in the lamina propria. These form a complex integrated network that responds to any noxious substance. The liver is part of the barrier function of the gut, since all toxins not eliminated by the gut reach this organ via the portal system and have to be detoxified by Phase I and Phase II enzymes.

Immune stimulation results in the release of chemical mediators, enzymes, oxidants and neurotransmitters, many of which affect epithelial function. Neurotransmitters can also stimulate or inhibit ion transport. The autonomic nervous system endings often appear in close relation to certain immune cells, such as mast cells in the lamina propria. Histamine from the latter (cells) activates the neural network to secrete ions into the lumen. Thus, to ward off noxious substances, the gut mucosa responds in a complex highly integrated fashion - hence dysregulation is ALL too simple.

Secretory IgA provides a line of defence against bacteria, food residue, fungus and yeast's, parasites and viruses. It neutralises invaders and prevents them from attaching to membranes. Deficiency of sIgA is a common immuno-deficiency and low-levels predispose to infections, asthma, autoimmune states, food allergies, candidiasis and coeliac disease etc. including Crohn's disease and ulcerative colitis. When high levels of sIgA are demonstrated they are the 'overload' of the immune system as in chronic viral conditions i.e. herpes sp, cytomegalo virus, Epstein-Barr virus and maybe Coxsachiae virus species, all of which tend to result in Chronic Fatigue Immunodeficiency Syndrome (CFIDS, ME, PVS etc.).

2.6.2

Causes of Increased Intestinal Permeability	
Prolonged use of nonsteroidal anti-inflammatory drugs (NSAID's)	AIDS
Chronic stress	Gastrointestinal disease
Dysbiosis	Immune overload
Environmental contamination / toxic substances	Deficiency of secretory IgA
Ageing	Overuse of alcoholic beverages
Food allergies and sensitivities	Trauma
Endotoxins	Chronic infections / presence of pathogenic bacteria, parasites and yeast
Chemotherapy / radiation therapy	

after Lipski

2.6.2.1 NSAID's, like ibuprofen and indomethacin deserve special mention as a particular specific causation of leaky-gut syndrome. They block prostaglandin's, including those which are used for healing and repair and those necessary for day to day repair of the gut lining, and may contribute to duodenitis and ulcerative colitis.

2.6.2.2 Antibiotics are also singled out for special mention and not just the medication ones, but those as residue in meats, poultry etc. Thus the territory is open to bacteroides, parasites, viruses, fungi (including Candida, where it exhibits a reaction antibody in 53-66% of all asthmatics tested. This could well be the result of steroid therapy, well known as a stimulator of Candida growth. Another factor may be low IgA subsequent to the asthma).

2.6.2.3 Other steroid factors in the treatment of allergies, autoimmune states, inflammatory states and emergency situations. These steroids (including topically applied) if used long-term will encourage candidiasis.

2.6.2.4 The hepatic overload is a serious state. The Phase I p450 Cytochrome system is stressed and results in the mixed function oxidases and causes depletion of their cofactors i.e. B vitamins, iron, zinc, copper and manganese. The Phase II sulphur containing amino-acids, methionine, cysteine, glycine and glutathione become depleted, as they are not regenerated during detoxification. Thus the body is deficient in these antioxidants and, hence, acetaldehyde and other undesirable metabolites get into the bloodstream (certainly during alcohol intake) and such then interfere at brain level. This results in cognitive dysfunction and chronic fatigue. Lipid peroxidation proceeds unabated by free radical scavengers.

The denatured proteins become under immune system influence and autoimmune system states ensue, together with other degenerative conditions. Chemical sensitivities follow as the liver's ability to cope with exo- and endotoxins (histamines, inflammatory metabolites etc.), especially to environmental inhalants or ingestants is impaired.

2.6.3 Protocols for 'Leaky Gut Syndrome'

Do You Have Leaky Gut Syndrome?

The following leaky gut syndrome questionnaire doesn't provide a definitive diagnosis, but it can help you assess the functioning of your small intestine. It is not intended to replace a physician's care or an intestinal permeability test. However, if you score high on this self-test, seek a physician who is knowledgeable about leaky gut to help you.

0 = Symptom is not present or rarely present
1 = Mild / sometimes
2 = Moderate / often
3 = Severe / almost always

INTESTINAL PERMEABILITY / LEAKY GUT SYNDROME, DYSBIOSIS

Constipation and / or diarrhoea	0	1	2	3
Abdominal pain or bloating	0	1	2	3
mucus or blood in stool	0	1	2	3
Joint pain or swelling, arthritis	0	1	2	3
Chronic or frequent fatigue or tiredness	0	1	2	3
Food allergies, sensitivities or intolerance	0	1	2	3
Sinus or nasal congestion	0	1	2	3
Chronic or frequent inflammations	0	1	2	3
Eczema, skin rashes or hives (urticaria)	0	1	2	3
Asthma, hayfever or airborne allergies	0	1	2	3
Confusion, poor memory or mood swings	0	1	2	3
Use of nonsteroidal antiimflammatory drugs (aspirin, Tylenol, Motrin)	0	1	2	3
History of antibiotic use	0	1	2	3
Alcohol consumption or alcohol makes you feel sick	0	1	2	3
Ulcerative colitis, Crohn's disease or celiac disease	0	1	2	3
Total:				

Score 1-5: Leaky gut less apt to be present.
Score 6-10: Leaky gut may possibly be present.
Score 11-19: Leaky gut probably present.
Score 20+: Leaky gut almost certainly present.

from Lipski 'Leaky Gut Syndrome'

Probable etiological flow chart for enhanced permeability

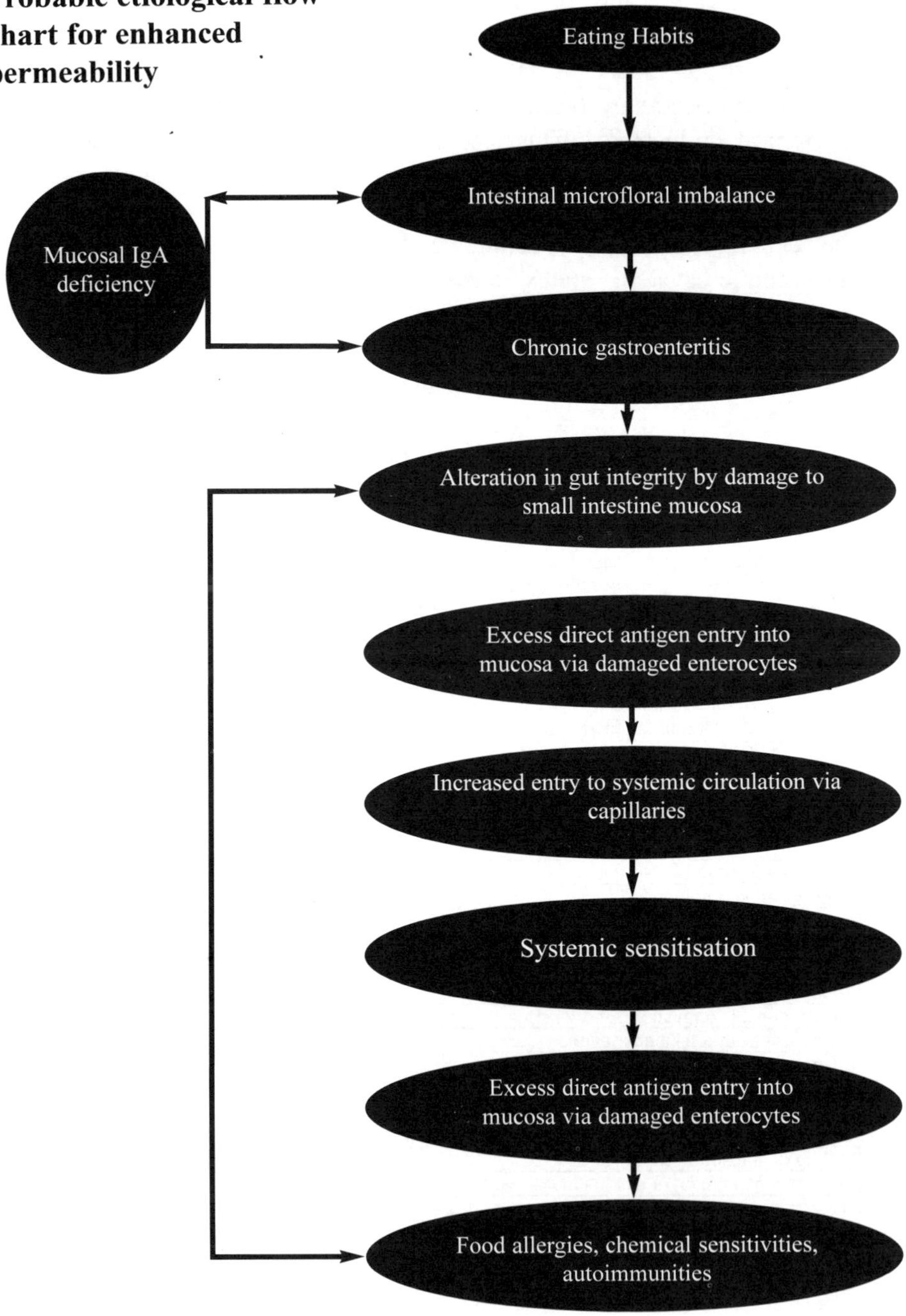

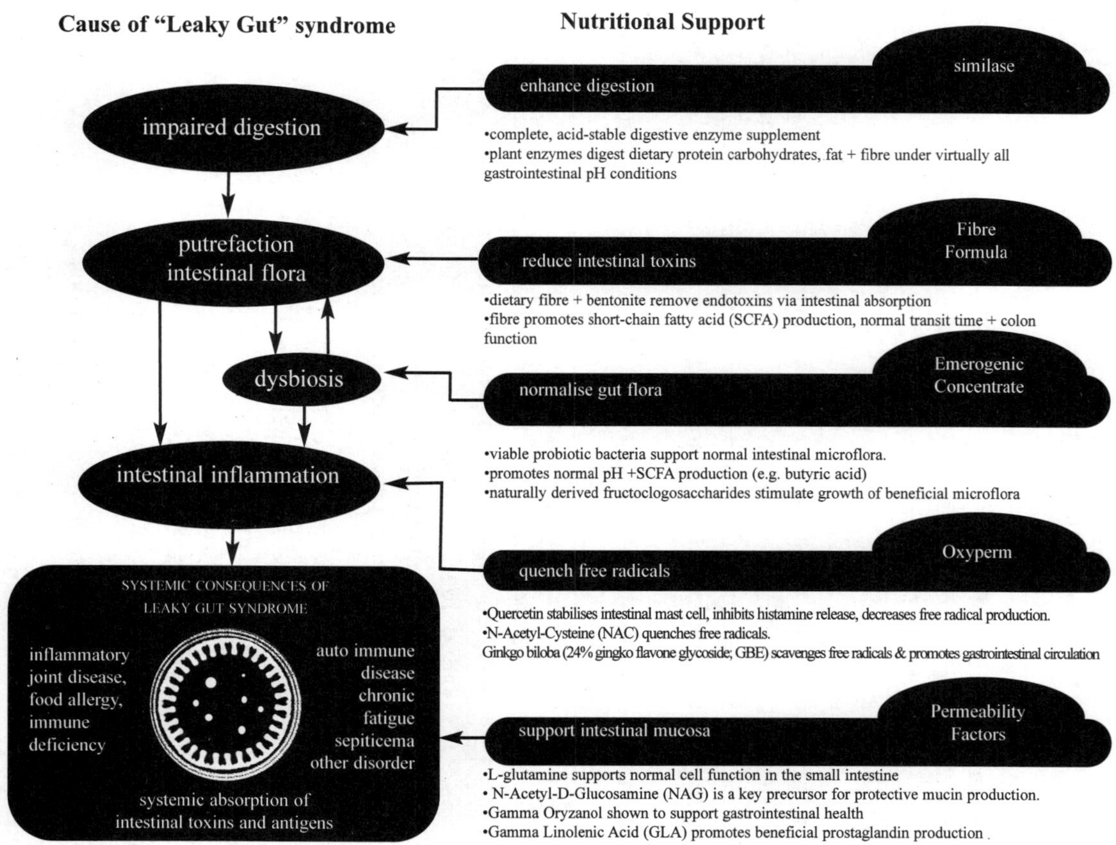
Cause of "Leaky Gut" syndrome
Nutritional Support
impaired digestion
putrefaction intestinal flora
dysbiosis
intestinal inflammation
SYSTEMIC CONSEQUENCES OF LEAKY GUT SYNDROME
inflammatory joint disease, food allergy, immune deficiency
auto immune disease chronic fatigue sepiticema other disorder
systemic absorption of intestinal toxins and antigens
enhance digestion
similase
•complete, acid-stable digestive enzyme supplement
•plant enzymes digest dietary protein carbohydrates, fat + fibre under virtually all gastrointestinal pH conditions
reduce intestinal toxins
Fibre Formula
•dietary fibre + bentonite remove endotoxins via intestinal absorption
•fibre promotes short-chain fatty acid (SCFA) production, normal transit time + colon function
normalise gut flora
Emerogenic Concentrate
•viable probiotic bacteria support normal intestinal microflora.
•promotes normal pH +SCFA production (e.g. butyric acid)
•naturally derived fructoclogosaccharides stimulate growth of beneficial microflora
quench free radicals
Oxyperm
•Quercetin stabilises intestinal mast cell, inhibits histamine release, decreases free radical production.
•N-Acetyl-Cysteine (NAC) quenches free radicals.
Ginkgo biloba (24% gingko flavone glycoside; GBE) scavenges free radicals & promotes gastrointestinal circulation
support intestinal mucosa
Permeability Factors
•L-glutamine supports normal cell function in the small intestine
• N-Acetyl-D-Glucosamine (NAG) is a key precursor for protective mucin production.
•Gamma Oryzanol shown to support gastrointestinal health
•Gamma Linolenic Acid (GLA) promotes beneficial prostaglandin production .

2.6.3.1 Leaky Gut Syndrome Management

Aim - to Overcome:
1) Inflammation and allergy
2) Malabsorption
3) Hepatic overload
4) Dysbiosis

Then the repair of the intestinal mucosa is undertaken. The 4-R approach of Eleanor BARRAGER of Health comm International seems favourite, together with a programmed enjoy healthy eating (FSA) behavioural eating habit modification regime. I have modified the 4-R system slightly.

A. Remove i.e. the dysbiosis - probably involving Candida protocol below.
Parasite seeking and removal.
Enteropathogen seeking and removal.
Food intolerance and removal (see relevant section).
Refined sugar, refined white flour products, alcohol, yeast based food, caffeine, NSAID, antibiotic and saturated fat removal and avoidance.
Detoxification procedures - see later.

B. Replace
1) Digestive enzymes HCl, plant derived proteases, amylases, lipases, cellulases.
2) Antioxidants.
3) Total nutrient intake - i.e. 6 grams daily Chlorella, Spirulina, Aloe Vera.
4) Sulphur amino-acid supplements.

C. Reinoculate and Replenish - basically probiotics - see Part IV.

D. Repair
1) Vitamins - B group, B5, Vit C, B12
2) Minerals - Zinc, Selenium, Iron.
3) Omega 6 and Omega 3 essential fatty acids.
4) Gradual introduction of dietary fibre (NSP) starting with pectins, gums and mucilages.
5) FOS supplementation - see Dietary Fibre section.
6) Glutathione and N-acetyl cystein.
7) Rice bran oil - excellent mucosal healer.
8) Homoeopathic and Anti-Homotoxic preparations (see Heel Mucosa Compositum, Hepeel, Leptandra

Compositum (for pancreatic support), Traumeel). All after Anti-Homotoxic detoxification regime.

The Candidiasis regime protocol is similar.

1) A more rigorous exclusion diet initially (see specialist books) with increased organic vegetables, olive oil usage, lots of garlic, unsmoked antibiotic, steroid and growth hormone free meat and poultry, linseed (flax) or Argan oil daily, fresh fruit and vegetable juice, chloride/fluoride free water.

2) Use Nystatin if serious infestation for one week ONLY.
   " Caprylic acid - coconut extract
   " Garlic capsules
   " Tried and tested herbs - Astragalus, Chaparral, Quassia, Fenugreek, Red sage, Black cohosh, Golden seal.

3) Metabolic cleansing regimes (see specialist books).

4) Eliminate herbicides, pesticides, food additives.

5) Establish healthy eating/drinking - mineral water.

6) Continue probiotic supplementation for at least 6 month and use vaginal probiotic pessaries.

7) Reduce environmental toxic effects - physical, chemical, biological.

8) Manage lifestyle stress a) embark graded exercise programme.

2.7 Dysbiosis - Irritable Bowel Syndrome (IBS)

(with acknowledgement to Paul Yanick Jr. Ph.D.)

2.7.1 IBS has many features of Leaky Gut Syndrome, indeed both may be present at the same time. Sufferers experience constipation and/or diarrhoea or may continually alternate from one to the other; and stress results from the condition as also nutrient losses, sometimes resulting in low grade malnutrition of 'key nutrients' e.g. Vitamin B12. There are undoubtedly associated conditions which may be primary or secondary. D[r] Yanick names duodenitis as primary - possibly from Helicobacter pylori causation, with oral presence of the bacterium perhaps being its 'niche' location.

Dysbiosis certainly is present but, again, whether primary or secondary is variant pathology. Certainly, also, IBS is probably a resultant of dysregulation of the extracellular matrix of Reckeweg/Pischinger with interference of normal lymph flow.

2.7.2 IBS has multifactorial causation and cases vary as to the predominant factor:

1) **pH changes in GI Tract**
This basically is the tendency towards acidity, which of course may be dietary in origin i.e. too great an intake of animal protein, with too little raw vegetable greens etc. This is reflected in the common finding in IBS cases of a more acid bile - this may be a factor in the duodenitis, together with the Helicobacter pylori infection (it thrives in an acid environment).

2) **Duodenitis** - this certainly contributes to certain features of IBS i.e. bloating and flatulence, and gallbladder. As a result of this infection the lymph channels initially become overactive, but later 'clog up' and become permeable to gut toxins and low grade infections.

3) **Pleomorphic infections and Endotoxins** - these come from various foci, including dental, and from continuous low grade inflammation products and from the bacteria themselves. Such 'pleomorphs' probably 'leak' into the blood stream (? Are they the 'bodies' Enderlein and others find utilising dark-phase microscopy of blood - many could be yeast-like bodies?). Certainly, if such persist and progress, then sepsis ensues and, if antibiotics are used to get rid of the body's Helicobacter pylori, then multiple resistance may develop; allergies certainly do, necrosis of tissue may ensue, and perhaps viruses, especially Coxsachiae species are free to proliferate; and perhaps tumours.

The diagram on the next page gives some ideas of the parameters of neuro-hormonal dysregulation in regulation in relation to oestrogen dominance, and thyroid hormones.

4) **Neuro-hormonal dysregulation** - this is a complex and broad spectrum of effects. It certainly involves the pituitary hypothalamic axis (shades of Reckeweg's Homotoxicology again) and probably involves the thyroid (low output) and the thymus gland (monitor of the immune system via its 4 hormones and recently found to have autonomic nervous system input), and immune system factors need to be considered concomitantly.

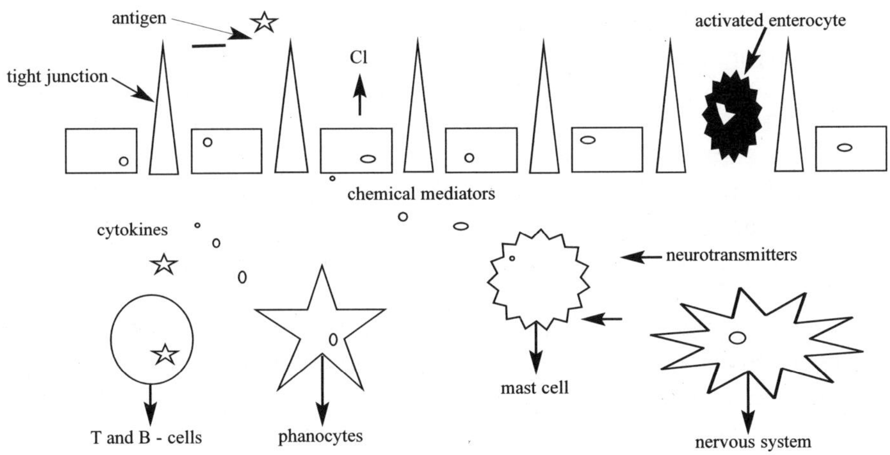

2.7.3 The influence of GALT, both inwardly and outwardly is most important in respect of dysbiosis and its effects, especially in IBS. It appears that the duodenitis results in maldigestion, which in turn results in allergic inflammatory responses to the undigested food particulates. These in turn react with the GALT and the gut flora to produce an immunological response which tends to affect the villi and nutrient absorption. Now, we already know and have seen the GALT neuro-endocrine links via the messenger biological molecules i.e. cytokines, prostaglandin's and neuropeptides. Thus further pro-inflammatory cytokines are released and the cycle continues in a downward spiral and is compounded by a more acidic gut pH. Dysbiosis ensues or becomes more disrupted.

Thus, management protocols become self-evident:

A) Correct the duodenitis.

B) Return to general norm gut pH.

C) Detoxify using the principles of Anti-Homotoxic regime according to the Reckeweg system - see Annex; and including total liver/lymphatic detoxification by appropriate methods.

D) Remove anti-yeast, anti-fungal factors.

E) Synchronise or re-synchronise to improve the functional status and biological molecular communication system's of the body's bio-energetic physiological homeostatic systems, and fine-tune meridian energies (acupuncture).

F) Thus re-establish GALT integrity using probiotics, prebiotics and total optimal nutrient status in the gut micro-ecology and stabilise colonic mucosal function and exclude reactive oxygen and reactive nitrogen species, stress as also any heavy metal (mercury) toxicity.

2.7.4 N.B. In association with the above protocol, it is important to be aware of the electro-anatomy of the living organism (ref: What is Homotoxicology All About - article by Prof M.F. Kirkman).

This energy pattern can be measured today and used diagnostically and therapeutically. The energy anatomy requires nourishment in today's pollutant, toxic environment. Such can be attained by therapies that support the harmonic resonance of cells, tissues, glands and organs. Certainly, such concepts must include the GALT and the intestinal microflora (see Virtual Medicine, Dr Keith Scott-Mumby, Thorsons 2000 - foreword by Prof M.F. Kirkman).

The ultimate medicine must have the ability to control at the most fundamental level i.e. biological molecules, the biological life processes that give rise to health and healing. Again GALT and intestinal microbiological balance must be most important in this status quo; and Probiotic Therapy an integrated part of such thesis.

Bio-Energetic Medicine defines health as a function of proper alignment and balance internally and externally, co-ordination and balance of the meridian system and its related organs and systems of the body (including ground matrix regulation). The concept that human beings (to the author Homo electro magneticus) possess higher dimensional homeostatic systems (the cybernetic concept of von Bertolffi) that govern neuro-hormonal and immune bio-regulation is the main tenet underlying this approach.

This higher dimensional anatomy also determines structural patterning in the extra-cellular and cellular matrix of the physical body (which indicates the role and importance of a balanced intestinal flora influencing such via the GALT and bio-communicating molecules).

The body cannot just be seen as physical nerves, total and local hormones, muscles and bones, 21st century physicians MUST incorporate their beloved linear scientific logic and evidence based medicine concepts and view the body as a multidimensional being of energy whose physical body is but a single component of a larger dynamic system (Integrated Medicine Approach).

Because each organ (the intestinal GALT/microflora can be considered one such entity) within the body has its own resonant frequency supplying the body with both physical and energetic nourishment is of paramount importance (the reason the intestinal flora is so susceptible to electromagnetic, radiation and low frequency sound waves).

It is important to grasp, especially in the presence of dysbiosis and ensuing chronic and multifaceted illness, that the cells that compose our organ structures are nourished not only by oxygen, glucose and other nutrients, but also by streams of energy containing specific resonance frequencies that cause enzymes to function and give LIFE to the organism.

Part III : Clinical Protocols / Probiotics

3.1 Nature and role of probiotics

The author is grateful to Bernard Dugas, FRACTALES Biotech S.A., ACMO parc, 10 Ave de Reaumur 92140 Clamart, France; Annick Mercennier, Institute Pasteur de Lille, 59000 Lille, France; Irene Lenoir-Wijnkoop, Cecile Arnaud, Nathalie Dugas and Eric Postaire, Groupe Nutrition et Sante, CIRDC, 92270 Les Plessis Robinson, France.

Probiotics are living micro-organisms that promote the health of the host by improving the microflora. A recent meeting focused on the immunoregulatory properties of probiotics with the aim of identifying their cellular and molecular mechanisms of action.

Certain conditions when probiotics are of importance
Below there follows a variety of conditions, which are more or less related to dysbiosis. The dysbiotic condition is directly or indirectly related to symptoms.

Gastritis and ulcer
Gallbladder dysfunction and liver diseases
Irritable colon
Constipation or diarrhoea
Dyspepsia
Migraine; conversion of tyrosine to tyrosamine
Atopies i.e. eczema, hay fever, urticaria, asthma
Food intolerance i.e. gluten intolerance
Chronic inflammatory diseases or autoimmune diseases such as rheumatism, SLE, fibromyalgia, psoriasis, colitis ulcerosa, mb.Crohn etc.
Infections in the urinary system
Mycosis i.e. Candida albicans
Exposition to radiation, cortisone, antibiotics, contraceptives
Conditions with impaired immune defence i.e. malignant disease, leucemias
Insufficiency of vitamins or minerals
Skin disease i.e. acne, herpes
Stress
Hormonal dysfunction i.e. bleedings, menstruation dysfunction, infertility and osteoporosis
Metabolic syndrome and diabetes
Chronic fatigue syndrome and, possibly, Ankylosing spondylitis and Autism and post vaccination / inoculation states.

Suggested health effects of probiotics

1. Increased nutritional value (better digestibility, increases absorption of minerals and vitamins)
2. Promotion of intestinal lactose digestion
3. Positive influence on intestinal flora (antibiotics or radiation induced colitis)
4. Prevention of intestinal tract infections (bacteria or virus induced, Candida enteritis, Helicobacter pylori ulcus/neoplasia)
5. Regulation of gut motility (constipation, irritable bowel syndrome)
6. Improvement of immune system
7. Prevention of cancer
8. Reduction of catabolic products eliminated by kidney and liver
9. Prevention of atherosclerosis (reduction of serum cholesterol)
10. Prevention of osteoporosis
11. Better development (growth)
12. Improved well-being

3.1.2
Probiotics and colorectal cancer

As probiotics, the intestinal flora play an important role in the induction and development of colon cancer. However, the probiotic effect that remains the most controversial is the anticancer activity attributed to certain LAB. Two types of studies have been conducted in this field (J. Rafter, Huddinge): (1) *in vitro* and *in vivo* animal models studies; and (2) dietary intervention studies in humans and epidemiological studies correlating cancer to certain dietary regimes. Although there is no direct evidence that LAB prevent or protect humans from colon cancer, many indirect effects based on experimental animal models suggest a probiotic effect on colon cancer protection.

Mechanisms by which probiotics might inhibit colon cancer

- Suppress the growth of intestinal microflora incriminated in producing putative mutagens / carcinogens and promoters
- Produce antimutagenic and antitumourigenic compounds in the colon
- Bind potential mutagens and carcinogens
- Alter physiological conditions in the colon (lowering the pH) affecting the metabolic activity of the intestinal flora, the action of bile acids and causing quantitative and / or qualitative alterations in the bile acid degrading bacteria
- Enhance the host's immune sys tem

3.1.3 Probiotics and Diarrhoea

Different randomised, controlled clinical trials have demonstrated that Lactobacillus rhamnosis GG with L casei DN-114001 (LC) is effective in the treatment of gastro-enteritis, especially in the case of infantile rotavirus diarrhoea (Isolauri; P. Reinert, Creteil). In the group of infants receiving GG, levels of IgC, IgA and IgM increased temporarily. More strikingly cells secreting anti-rotavirus IgA were observed at much higher numbers than in the control group, leading to protection against re-infection.

3.1.4 Probiotics and allergy

The immune system of the elderly is well established but weakens with ageing, whereas in babies or young infants the intestinal tract, which is sterile at birth, becomes progressively populated with different bacterial species. The role of the gut microflora in the maturation of the mucosal immune barrier is well recognised and can best be seen in new-borns. The latter are rapidly exposed to foreign antigens after birth when delivered by the vaginal route (maternal bacterial flora) and breast fed (food antigens). After about one year, the immune system starts to establish tolerance. In some cases, an atopic status characterised by high (excessive) IgE responses can occur and this normally reverses spontaneously to tolerance. However, a quarter of young children develop multiple food allergy, a so-called 'atopic -disease'. In babies, atopic eczema or dermatitis occurs along with intestinal disorders, leading to a reduced growth rate.

The classical treatment of this disease consists of eliminating the incriminated antigen of the food source (elimination diets), which may prove very inconvenient from a practical point of view. In addition, immunotherapy and stabilisation of the gut microflora and mucosa can be attempted. Clinical studies have been conducted on infants developing dermatitis or cow's milk allergy to evaluate if LAB probiotic strains could prevent or reduce allergic symptoms; the *in vivo* (faecal) level of tumour necrosis factor (TNF-a) is strongly reduced. Additional immunological parameters that reflect the Th1 / Th2 balance were measured demonstrating reduced intestinal inflammation. This study is an example of a well-conducted clinical trial proving that selected LAB strains can exert a healthy effect in the context of neonatal allergy.

3.1.5 Some Probiotics (in addition to the standard Lactic Acid Bacteria Bifidobacteria Acidophilus species)

a. **Lactobacillus plantarum**

Of the various lactobacilli found to inhabit the colon as part of the indigenous flora Lactobacillus plantarum has a number of positive attributes. Its name plantarum has the same origin as the word 'plant' and it is found throughout the vegetable kingdom. It is found throughout the food we eat daily, in particular fermented vegetables, on greens, fish and in the brine of olives. Lactobacillus plantarum is essential for the development of a favourable flavour and smell in sauerkraut, the brine of dill cucumber (Wyss and Eklund) and some cheeses especially the hard varieties. The total count of lactobacilli and streptococci, both dead and alive is extremely large and probably accounts for as much as 0.1 per cent of the weight of the cheese (Hawker and Linton). It has been suggested that part of L plantarum's beneficial activity can be attributed to its very high production of lactic acid and of the essential amino acid lysine and methionine (over 500 times greater than other strains of L plantarum - University of Montana U.S.A. 1988). Lysine has been found to have a number of therapeutic effects and is known in helping to control the herpes simplex virus accompanied by a diet low in arginine. Methionine is also of therapeutic value, for example, as a free radical scavenger and is effective for eliminating toxic metals from the body (Chaitow 1985).

b. **Streptococcus lactis**

Streptococcus lactis is found in many dairy products, cheeses and butter. It is naturally occurring in foods and is one of the organisms which sours raw milk, in doing so it ferments the lactose content of the milk. In the body Streptococcus lactis is also found in the indigenous flora and colonises higher regions in the gastrointestinal tract such as the mouth and oesophagus.

c. **Streptococcus faecium**

Streptococcus faecium is found as part of the indigenous flora in a healthy colon. The strain of Streptococcus faecium in symbiotic bacteria has been carefully selected for its properties from the thousands of other possibilities. The anti-microbial properties of Streptococcus faecium are well documented in the scientific literature. It is noted for its action against salmonella and other enteropathogens as well as its ability to help liver functions and reduce levels of ammonia and other undesirable metabolites in the blood.

3.1.6 Probiotic Applications

by Mark A. Brudnak, PhD, ND

Probiotics: Viable single or mixed culture of micro-organisms which when applied to animal or human, beneficially affects their host by improving the properties of the indigenous microflora. Probiotics have found application in a wide variety of products including, yoghurt, dietary supplement capsules, tablets, milk, butter, cheese, salami, soy sauce, sour dough. They are even being used as anti-microbials for the poultry industry due to their ability to inhibit salmonella growth in chickens.

Probiotics are clearly here to stay and the market, despite its incredible growth over the last few years, is still in its infancy. Presently, there are identifiable trends in the use of probiotics. These trends can be generalised as a heightened awareness of differing quality in the organisms. From the manufacturing side, that includes such things as production of well-documented, clinically-backed strains, ability to survive gastric acid and bile salts, adherence, long-term stability. Also issues such as milk/casein-free are important for consumers.

Ten years ago, most probiotic products contained either Lactobacillus acidophilus or Bifidobacterium lactis (bifidum). If one was really lucky, they could find a combination of the two and possibly a couple of yoghurt strains (i.e., Lactobacillus bulgariucus) thrown in. Many of these contain only a few hundred million viable cells at the time of manufacture. While that may sound like a lot of organisms, especially when we are conditioned to think of bacteria as being 'bad', current data tells us that those numbers were probably far too low to be doing very much good. At least in the short-term, therapeutic application of the probiotics.

As more and more data comes in, it is becoming apparent that at least a billion organisms are needed per dose to achieve any real clinical significance. In a recent study, ten billion Bifidobacterium in milk per day were given and immune markers measured. A significant increase in phagocytic activity of granulocytes was observed.

In a randomised, double-blind placebo controlled study, the prophylactic effects of probiotics on infections in neutropenic patients undergoing cytoreductive chemotherapy for acute leukaemia was studied. Thirty patients (35 episodes) were included in the study. The lactobacilli were given as capsules thrice daily for 30 days, starting at the initiation of chemotherapy. The occurrence of fever was significantly (P=0.033, Mann-Whitney rank sum test) postponed from a median time of 8 days to 12 days. Capsules contained 50/50 Bifidobacterium lactis/lactobacillus acidophilus containing 4 billion/capsule.

In addition to immune parameters, the reduction of circulating ammonia has also been observed by Deguchi et al, using 5 billion organisms of either B lactis or B breve in caecal contents. They also observed a corresponding drop in the pH of the caecal contents. This lends support for the use of probiotics in detoxification protocols, which has been reported elsewhere.

Probiotic supplementation has been demonstrated to be very safe and effective for a wide variety of disturbances including antibiotic side effects, diarrhoea/constipation, lactose malabsorption and cholesterol reduction. Dosages ranging from one to almost 500 billion organisms have been used without complications. Current trends seem to indicate a range of 10-100 billion live organisms as being efficacious for the variety of conditions being mentioned above. At least two different companies have 'high-dose' products on the market with 20 and 30 billion organisms per capsule. These products should serve as a portent for the market as they were both originally designed for different markets, the environmentally challenged and autism (and Down's syndrome), respectively. These are excellent demonstrations of two principles that are developing. First, is a need for high-dose probiotics to treat selective conditions. Second, is the need for a variety of products.

What we are learning is that while a low-dose run-of-the-mill L acidophilus (providing it is well produced) can be great for a general maintenance program, oftentimes a much higher dose is required to achieve clinical significance. Additionally, it is becoming increasingly apparent that the inclusion of other strains, such as Lactobacillus rhamnosus or Lactobacillus plantarum (an exciting up-and-coming star) can have dramatic effect. The inclusion of multiple strains is not only beneficial for the specific conditions, but also may play another important role in the application of probiotics.

As can be seen, the area of probiotics is still in its infancy. This neonate is soon to grow-up, however, as major pharmaceutical companies enter this exciting and efficacious area of health care. As clinical data from the application of probiotics to conditions such as autism, downs syndrome, cancer, lactose intolerance, etc., comes to light, consumer/patient demand and awareness of the importance of these organisms, will concomitantly increase. With that, we can expect better products, tailored to specific conditions, to also be developed.

3.2 Probiotic Prescribing

INTESTINAL MICROBIOLOGY AND PROBIOTICS

Lennart Cedgard / MD assisted by Anna Kannius / Bsc in Biomedicine

Introduction

Probiotics have been defined as a live microbial feed supplement that beneficially influences the health of the host by improving the intestinal microflora. The use of probiotic bacteria in therapy is not a new invention. Yoghurt, containing probiotic bacteria have for hundreds of years been appreciated been appreciated for its health bringing properties.

Today, research is ongoing throughout the world to clarify the mechanisms of probiotics. Intake of probiotic bacteria have many positive effects on health like increasing the digestion and absorption of nutrients, improvement of intestinal lactose digestion, improving the intestinal milieu, regulating the gut motility, stimulating the immune system, prevention of cancer, reduction of catabolic products eliminated by kidney and liver etc.

The concepts of Metchnikoff 1908 are thus finally being confirmed both experimentally and clinically. Metchnikoff (1845 - 1916) claimed in his theory of longevity that intake of yoghurt decreases the toxic effect of the colonic flora by inhibiting the growth of putrefactive bacteria in the large intestine. He further claimed that the toxic products produced by putrefactive bacteria are the cause of many ageing processes in the body and that the long life of Bulgarian peasants resulted from their consumption of fermented milk products. Continuous conditioning of the intestinal ecosystem is useful in medicine and routine care, particularly in aged individuals.

Why is there a need of probiotic bacteria today?

In modern times, we have dramatically changed the consumption of bacteria entering our body via food and drinks. The intake of bacteria, preferably *Lactobacillus* species is highly reduced. In former times, fermentation was one of the main ways of preserving food, vegetables and dairy products. This assured a constant intake of lactic acid-producing bacteria. Today the situation has changed. Use of freezers, refrigerators and pasteurisation of feeds like dairy products and the use of different kinds of preservatives have replaced fermentation as a method for preservation of food. Today, most people do not get probiotic bacteria via the food in the same amount as former times. As a matter of fact we almost dont get ant bacteria at all. Use of antibiotics in health care and agriculture, and the increased hygienic measures in modern society with antibacterial substances in cleaning agents, toothpaste, deodorants etc., have decreased the amount of total bacteria in our environment. Studies have shown differences between the intestinal microflora of people in developed and developing countries, both in infants (2) (3) and adults (26). In developing countries, people have a more varied intestinal microflora with more strains and a higher turnover of bacteria. In Western industrialised countries we have relatively few strains in the intestinal flora and we keep the strains for longer periods, maybe years. A high turnover of bacteria is certainly important in keeping the immune system stimulated (39).

On top of this, we have today a higher pressure on the bacterial ecosystem in our body than in old times through a changed diet (rich in protein, fat and refined products like sugar and poor in fibres), stress, increased intake of medicines like antibiotics, and environmental toxins etc. The need of probiotic bacteria is thus due to the many factors in our society that can damage the intestinal health and the fact that the intake of probiotic bacteria via the food has decreased. A healthy intestinal milieu is crucial for our health.

We have, since the discovery of bacteria and the invention of antibiotics, had the general idea that the major part of the microbes are pathogenic but it is in fact only a minor part of the thousands of bacterial species that are harmful to humans.

Ecological Background

The intestinal microflora

There is a whole world of 'micro life' in our intestines. The normal intestinal microflora build up a fantastic ecosystem, which is extremely complex and impossible to understand completely. What we know today is that our intestinal microflora consists of about 10^{14} cells, which is ten times the number of human cells in our body. The normal microflora, sometimes called the biggest 'organ' in the body has a weight of approximately 0.5 - 1.0kg and at present it is estimated to consist of 400 different species. However, recent genetic research shows that, when mapping the genome of the colonic bacteria only 35 percent could be identified and assigned to known bacteria. The remainder were unknown!

The stomach and the upper part of the small intestine contain low counts of bacteria (10^3 - 10^5/ml gastric juice) due to the gastric- and bile acid.

Further down in the small intestine the number of bacteria increase to 10^6 - 10^7 and in the colon the counts are as high as 10^{11}/g faeces.

The intestinal microflora consists of both aerobic bacteria, which need oxygen to survive, and anaerobic bacteria that will die in the presence of oxygen. There are also facultative anaerobic bacteria, which can live in both aerobic and anaerobic milieus. Immediately after birth, bacteria start colonising the skin and mucosal membranes like the respiratory tract and the intestine. During the first few days of life the milieu in the intestine is rich in oxygen. Therefore the first colonisers are aerobic and facultative anaerobic bacteria like E.coli and other Enterobacteriaceae, Enterococcus spp and Staphylococcus spp. (6) (7) (36). When these bacteria start proliferating they consume oxygen so the intestinal milieu will become more and more anaerobic, which in turn makes it possible for anaerobic bacteria like Bacteroides, Bifidobacterium, Clostridium and Lactobacillus to start colonising. Within a few days anaerobic bacteria will dominate the intestinal microflora of the infant and in adults more than 99% of the bacteria in the intestine are anaerobic. The intestinal microflora of infants are much simpler and much more liable to fluctuate than the one of the adults, which is generally very 'stable'. During the wea ning period the infants bacterial flora starts to resemble the one of the adult but may not be fully developed until 4-8 years of age.

The dominant species in an adult's colon are Bacteroides and Bifidobacterium whereas the small intestine is dominated by Lactobacillus spp and Streptococcus spp. It is possible that the flora in the proximal parts of the gastrointestinal tract, though quantitatively much smaller than that in the colon, is most important since its products pass the absorptive part of the intestine. The bacteria in the small intestine may also have the strongest influence on the immune system since the gut-associated-lymphoid-tissue (GALT) is situated mainly in the small intestinal wall.

Some bacteria are said to be colonising, which means that they are able to colonise, proliferate and remain in the intestine for longer periods, weeks, months or years. Other bacteria are referred to as transient. These bacteria enter the gastrointestinal tract via food or drinks and are in transit from the mouth to the anus. They are not colonising the gastrointestinal tract, but contribute to about 30% of the faecal weight.

The habitats of the normal bacterial flora in the intestine are shredded intestinal cells or food particles, the mucosa, or rather the overlying mucous layer and the Lieberkuhn's crypts. The crypts have shown to contain a very specific flora, often consisting of a single species. Both the cryptflora and the mucosal flora may be physiologically important but not reflected in faecal cultures. Another fact to consider is that the cell turnover may be great although the culture counts are not impressive.

Even though the intestinal flora of adults are considered as stable considering the composition of the species, new strains are entering the intestinal tract all the time via food and beverages or in other ways swallowed, and other strains leave via the faeces. Thus there is a constant turnover of bacteria in the intestine, which is very important for the stimulation of the immune system.

In 1972 van der Waaij introduced the term 'competitive colonisation' which describes the interference between the normal intestinal microflora and the invading pathogens. By competing for nutrients and space and by secretion of antibacterial substances the normal intestinal microflora can prevent pathogenic bacteria from colonising. In a germ free animal only 10-100 salmonella bacteria are needed for infection to occur while in a conventional animal it takes 1,000,000 bacteria. The prerequisite for a bacterial infection to occur is that the normal microflora is disturbed.

The intestinal ecology is vital in both the genesis, prevention and treatment of disease.

The small intestine and the immune system

The mucosal membrane of the intestine, which has an area of around 200m^2, is under constant challenge by different kinds of antigens. Not only do we swallow food antigens (60-70 tons throughout a lifetime) and food-borne microbes, but also inhaled particles that become trapped in the respiratory tract and transported up the pharynx are finally swallowed and reach the intestine. Furthermore, the mucosal membrane of the intestine has intimate contact with the normal intestinal microflora. It is therefore not surprising that the intestine contains the largest accumulation of lymphoid tissues in the body. Eighty percent (!) Of the lymphocytes in the body are situated in the intestinal wall, in the so-called gut-associated-lymphoid-tissue (GALT). They appear as aggregates in lymph nodules called Peyer's patches and as scattered lymphoid cells in the lamina propria. Further, the intestinal epithelia are seeded by small lymphocytes termed intraepithelial lymphocytes. The GALT is associated with the rest of the lymphatic system via lymphatic vessels directed toward lymph nodules situated in the mesenteric fibrous tissue that lines the small intestine.

The immune system has two major functions, equally important: to react to foreign, dangerous antigens and particles like pathogenic bacteria and viruses and to *not* react on harmless antigens like food antigen and body tissue. These two functions have shown to be associated with each other.

Intestinal immune responses to bacteria are mainly induced in the Peyer's patches. When lymphocytes (B- and T-cells) in the Peyer's patches are activated by bacterial antigens they start to proliferate and leave the intestinal tissue for the blood. They circulate for a couple of days before they settle down somewhere in the mucosal-associated-lymphoid-tissue (MALT) (10) (31) (16), which is the lymphoid tissue associated with all the mucosal membranes in the body like the intestinal, respiratory and uro-genital mucosa. Lymphoid tissues of all the mucosal membranes in the body are in this way interconnected. Immunological reactions, like allergic reactions in the intestine are likely to influence the status of other mucosal tissues. (These findings can be connected to old knowledge telling that 'the intestine is the mother of the lung'). When the activated B -cells have settled down they mature and start producing IgA antibodies. Thus, the bacteria induce immunity against themselves. The paradox is that at the same time as the bacteria induce strong immunological reactions against themselves, they decrease immunological reactivity against other antigens like food antigens. The mechanism of this is not completely known, but studies have shown that it is difficult to achieve oral tolerance in animals lacking an intestinal microflora (28) (42) while administration of bacterial antigens with the food increases the tolerising effect of feeding (20). Conversely some bacterial toxins like cholera toxin may break oral tolerance to food antigens (12) so the composition of the intestinal flora is of importance.

Further, studies point to the importance of a high turnover of bacteria for the stimulation of the immune system. It is important that the immune system meets with new bacterial antigens continuously. As soon as IgA antibodies are produced against a certain bacterial antigen, antibodies bind to the antigen and inhibit it from translocating the intestinal wall and reaching the Peyer's patches (39). The low turnover of bacteria and the decreased number of bacterial strains in the intestinal microflora of people in the western world may lead to a decreased bacterial stimulation of the immune system which could lead to over-reactivity against other antigens like food antigens.

The immune system of an infant is not fully developed. The intestinal barrier is immature and the capacity to generate IgA producing cells is inadequate. Bacterial colonisation provides maturational signals to the GALT (17). Thus, the intestinal microflora is important for the maturation of the immune system in infants. Animals lacking an intestinal microflora have very small Peyer's patches, the level of IgA antibodies in the blood is low and the amount of T-cells in the intestinal wall is also decreased.

General aspects of probiotics

Probiotics have been defined as live microbial feed supplements that beneficially affect the host by improving the intestinal bacterial balance. Bacterial species commonly referred to as probiotic are lactic-acid producing bacteria such as Bifidobacterium spp, Lactobacillus spp and Streptococcus spp, but also other micro-organisms like the fungi S.boulardii have been used. There are many properties of probiotic bacteria that may help to improve the intestinal milieu like their metabolism, cell-wall structures and intracellular components.

Suggested beneficial effects of probiotics, as were published in 'Trends of immunology today' 1999, are:

- Increased nutritional value (better digestibility, increased absorption of minerals and vitamins).
- Promotion of intestinal lactose digestion.
- Positive influence on the intestinal microflora (antibiotics or radiation induced colitis).
- Prevention of intestinal tract infections (bacteria or virus induced, Candida enteritis, Helicobacter pylori ulcus/neoplasia).
- Regulation of gut motility.
- Improvement of the immune system.
- Prevention of cancer.
- Reduction of catabolic products eliminated by kidney and liver.
- Prevention of atherosclerosis by reduction of serum cholesterol.
- Prevention of osteoporosis.
- Better development (growth).
- Improved well-being.

Lactic-acid-producing bacteria metabolise nutrients by fermentation. During this process different organic acids are formed like (L+) lactic acid and butyric acid, which lowers the intestinal pH. The lowered pH has many beneficial effects on the intestinal milieu like inhibiting growth of putrefactive bacteria. Putrefactive bacteria produce nitrogen waste products during digestion of nutrients. The benefits of inhibiting growth of these bacteria are the reduction of blood ammonia, free serum phenols and free amino acids in the urine. This implies improved nitrogen retention. These characteristics could be responsible for the growth and improved body weight (muscle volume) seen in different animal studies. Reduced concentration of nitrogen related toxins play an important role in the detoxification of the liver. Uric acid, the natural antioxidant produced in the liver as a response to excess amounts of free radicals, is related to the level of dysbiosis in the intestinal tract. This explains why probiotics will stimulate liver regeneration and subsequently would be used in a 'liver support program'.

It is often claimed that a probiotic culture has to be able to adhere to the intestinal epithelia and colonise the intestine to have any effect. This issue is controversial. First of all, what is the definition of a 'colonising bacteria' ? Colonising bacteria are sometimes referred to as bacteria that are more permanently found in an individuals flora but in other cases as bacteria remaining in the intestinal flora for 1-3 days are considered as colonising (15). In constipated people transient bacteria can probably be found in faeces for longer periods than three days.

A method often used to test a bacteria's ability to colonise in the intestine is to see if they adhere to intestinal epithelial cells in vitro. This is not a fully adequate way of looking at colonisation ability since there are other habitats for colonising bacteria than the epithelia, like the overlying mucosal layer and loose particles. Thus, bacteria with negative results in the test mentioned may still be able to colonise. Ninety-nine percent of the intestinal microflora consists of anaerobic bacteria which means that they die in the presence of oxygen. The area closest to the epithelia is probably not the preferable habitat for these bacteria since oxygen diffuses from underlying blood vessels to the epithelial cells and then to the supraepithelial area. This supports the fact that bacteria must not be able to adhere to the intestinal epithelia to be able to colonise. Lactobacillus GG have been shown to reduce both travellers diarrhoea, antibiotic-associated diarrhoea and relapsing Clostridium difficile colitis even though only 'colonising' for 1 -3 or 7 days, which in some cases are considered as transient.

Bacterial strains regarded as transient can certainly also have effect when administered in high counts by interaction with the immune system and by improving the intestinal environment, stimulating growth of the normal bacterial flora.

Nutritional aspects of probiotics

All mineral- and vitamin substitution will demand a healthy intestinal ecosystem. The microflora must be in good shape and in balance for the nutritional system to be able to effectively take in and utilise minerals and vitamins. This is often not the case. The metabolism of proteins, lipids and carbohydrates will improve if the bacterial flora is in balance. Some new alimentary and pharmaceuticals, stress of different origins influence our bodies in many biological levels. The endocrine, the immune and the nutritional system are dependent that both the external and the internal ecology are in balance.

Daily conditioning with probiotics are to be seen as a supplementation of friendly bacteria that we are supposed to get and that we did get earlier but not any longer due to modern techniques of preserving food.

All mineral- and vitamin supplementation demands a **Healthy intestinal ecosystem.**

The nutritional interactions between the probiotics and the host are:

Bacteria consume vitamins. When there is an overgrowth of colonic bacteria in the small intestine the loss of vitamins due to bacterial consumption can be remarkable and can lead to vitamin deficiency. Probiotic bacteria inhibits overgrowth of colonic bacteria in the small intestine and therefore reduces the loss of vitamins. Compare to imbalances in spite of additional intake of vitamins.

An improved effect on the mineral absorption due to:

- Osmotic effects
- Increased production of organic acids due to the fermentation and the production of short-chain carboxylic acids.
- Increased formation of soluble salts of these acids.
- Proliferation of the intestinal wall.

Enzyme induction or enzyme support will improve the absorption of nutrients.

Increased production of the vitamins B1, B2, B6, B12, nicotinic acid, folic acid and biotin from the stimulated bifidobacteria. These vitamins are absorbed by the intestine and utilised by the different tissues of the human body.

Reduced production of toxins or so-called free radicals, which consume vitamins, minerals and antioxidants, produced by the body itself i.e. uric acid.

To be noted: the most production of free radicals is to be seen in the intestine. This will increase if the microflora is dysbiotic. Bifidobacteria and lactobacilli produce organic acids, which will work as antioxidatives. Studies by (19) shows that there is a reduction of app. 70% of the oxidative activity in the intestine, which also implied a better status of vitamin E (35).

Immunological aspects of probiotics

Probiotics have been defined as live microbial feed supplements that beneficially affect the host by improving the intestinal bacterial balance. Probiotics have a stimulating effect on the immune system, both the innate and specific immunity. It is though important to notice that different probiotic bacteria may elicit different kinds of immunological responses. The administration route of bacteria is also important to consider when testing the immunological response to probiotics. Many bacterial species die during the pathway through the stomach and upper small intestine, which reduces the immunological effect of these bacteria. Using acid and bile acids resistant strains or by tabletting the bacteria assures that the main part of the supplemented bacteria reach the intestine and can be immunologically active.

The normal intestinal microflora is part of the innate immune system. By 'competitive colonisation' (43) commensal bacteria inhibit pathogenic bacteria from colonising the mucosal tissue which is the initial step of infection. Probiotic bacteria inhibit colonisation of pathogens by producing organic acids like lactic acid and butyric acid which lowers the intestinal pH and in that way inhibits growth of potentially pathogenic micro-organisms. They also produce other bactericins that inhibit the growth of certain bacteria. Competition for nutrients and space are also involved in the term competitive colonisation. The antimicrobial activity of probiotic bacteria explains the usefulness of such bacteria for conservation of food.

Regarding the influence of probiotics on the cell-mediated immunity, research has shown that intake of probiotic bacteria increase the production of IgA antibodies (18)(32)(27)(44), increase the activity of macrophages and NK-cells (34)(33)(5), which leads to an increased killing of bacteria. It has also been shown that probiotic bacteria modulate the cytokine activity. Cytokines are signal substances in the immune system, which regulate the activity of the immune cells. Probiotics stimulate the immune system in an 'antiallergic' direction with decreased production of IgE antibodies as a result (25). Cytokines also work as a link between the immune system and the nervous system.

The mucosa of the intestines is a selective barrier which, when functioning normally, prevents the penetration of potentially noxious agents into the bloodstream, while still enabling the passage of useful substances, such as nutrients, into the body fluids. The health of the intestinal wall is totally crucial for our health.

Probiotic bacteria also have a healing effect on the intestinal mucosal membrane by stimulation of the formation of epithelial cells and by decreasing inflammation in the intestine, shown by a decreased production of inflammatory cytokines during intake of probiotic bacteria [Mjamaa, 1997 #179]. A prerequisite for development of allergies is that substances, that in normal cases can not pass the intestinal barrier, leak out in the blood and come into contact with the immune system. It has been shown that atopic eczema is associated with intestinal inflammation (23) and increased antigen transfer over the intestinal barrier [Majamaa, 1996 #181]. The treatment of food allergies with probiotics has been shown to have positive effects (22).

Technical aspects of probiotics
As I have been involved for many years in the field of intestinal micro-ecology, my interest in how to develop probiotics has increased. There are some objectives that are to be looked upon if we are to create an 'optimal performance' probiotic product.

The choice of bacterial culture/s.
Would it be best with just one single strain culture or a mixture of different cultures? Some advocate that a multi-strain product is positive, due to being that there are different beneficial characteristics in the different cultures that will be added to each other. The performance of the different cultures can thus be synergistic (30). On the other hand it is more difficult to achieve high standards of quality control in such products. Single strain probiotics may be so far a little easier to document.

Quality and stability.
Freeze dried cultures are to be preferred. Tablets produced by low-compression method have a better stability than capsules.

Administration and packaging.
The freeze-dried powders would be packaged in an optimal form. To administer the powder itself directly into the gastrointestinal system is not specially cost effective. This is due to heavy losses directed by the bile acids and the stomach acids. These losses could be reduced by choosing acid tolerant and somewhat bile acid resistant cultures. Another way is to encapsulate the powder into gelatine capsules. The stability of the cultures is however influenced by the humidity in the gelatine!

Therefore many attempts have been made during the last few years to produce tablets. This is however quite difficult due to the compression that the bacteria cells will experience.

In the company Wasa medicals, where I am engaged, a new method of making tablets with viable cultures has been developed. This is a low compression method which minimises the split forces compared to conventional methods. The products benefiting from this technique are now intruding the market.

Probion is the first probiotic produced with a low compression technique using a unique and patent protected method, which makes it possible to manufacture the probiotic in a tablet form. This makes it possible to conduct the disintegration of the tablets in the gut, activating them properly in the right place and thereby achieving an optimal biological effect.

Background.
Tablets made with conventional methods will destroy cultures due to split and compression forces. Capsules consist of gelatine, most often made from animal fat and contain 10-15% water, which is detrimental to the cultures. This implies poor stability and viability. With powders administered in sachets or similar, it is difficult to control the exposure and disintegration in the intestinal tract and that will therefore reduce the effect of the cultures. The tablets give better storage, exposure and delivery. Research shows that customers (85%) prefer them.

Technology.
The method of tabletting has the advantage of promoting and improving the quality and the effect of the cultures, since it involves less compression, less split forces and reduced heat development. The cultures are protected in cavities formed during compression. The cultures are thus protected by mucus forming substances. This supports good viability and stability.

The tablet has a unique profile of disintegration (slow release), activating them completely in the right place and exposing them properly and for a longer period in the small intestine and thereby achieving an optimal biological effect. This is a difference compared to powders and capsules, where the disintegration is more direct and abrupt.

The patent involves the use of fructooligo- and polysaccharides. These are also defined as prebiotics and work in synergy with the probiotic cultures - synbiotics! The bacterial cultures will, by this formulation, get all the food they need to perform with an optimal effect.

Tablets make it easy to utilise the probiotics and other food supplements in a simple way, this will keep the system clean and optimise the absorption of food supplements. Probiotics must be seen as the primary food supplement.

Probion is to its definition probiotics + prebiotics = synbiotics, i.e. health promoting transient biocultures with influence on the gastrointestinal ecology. The probiotics work mainly through the substrate that the culture itself represents. As a complement to the probiotic cultures inulin acts as a substrate to the bifidobacteria. These metabolic fibres are considered prebiotics and contain fructooligosaccarides and fructopolysaccharides (FOS and FPS). They promote and stimulate the activities of the bifidobacteria and thus they are called bifidogenic.

Safety of probiotics

Probiotic cultures are 'generally recognised as safe' (GRAS). No case of infection has until now been traced to food-borne lactic acid-producing bacteria (1). However, theoretically all bacteria can become pathogens depending on the immunological status of the host so the safety of probiotic supplementation ought to be discussed.

Rare cases of local or systemic infections due to bifidobacteria, lactobacilli or other lactic acid-producing strains have been reported (13)(4)(14). However, in these cases nearly all patients were afflicted by a severe disease, like cancer or AIDS and most important, the infecting organism appeared to come from the patients own microflora. In two Finnish studies 9229 blood samples were cultured and the isolates were compared with dairy strains. Twenty samples contained lactobacilli, but none were identical to any of the commercial strains (38)(37). Theoretically, digestive lesions or immunodeficiency could increase the risk of infection caused by probiotic bacteria. However, S boulardii, a fungal probiotic has been given to patients with Crohn's disease with no side effects reported. Administration of probiotics have shown no immunological side effects like fever, arthritis or autoimmune diseases except for one case of autoimmune hepatitis that might have been enhanced by ingestion of large doses of yoghurt (9).

Diseases due to deleterious metabolic effects of probiotics have never been reported. However, supplementation of probiotics highly increases the number of bacteria in the small intestine, which could increase the deconjugation and dehydroxylation of bile acids to toxic, free secondary bile-salts. The biological effects of this have shown to be minimal (24) and it should not be considered as a dangerous side effect of the tested probiotic product.

Some probiotic bacteria have the ability to degrade mucus, which theoretically could harm the mucosal membrane of the intestine. A study of the mucous degrading effect of L.acidophillus, Bifidobacterium spp and L.rhamnosus showed no effect in vitro or in gnotobiotic rats mono associated with the strain.

Finally, the question of gene transfer. Antibiotic resistance genes, especially those carried by plasmids can be transferred between micro-organisms. The question is whether antibiotic resistance genes may be transferred between probiotic bacteria to pathogens and render them antibiotic resistant. It is well known that resistance to vancomycin can be transferred among E.faecium, which makes it important to investigate the safety of this strain. Some lactobacilli strains like L.casei, L.rhamnosus and L.plantarum are also resistant to vancomycin, but the resistance gene are chromosomally encoded and not transferable to pathogenic species. In conclusion the antibiotic resistance profile does not appear to be a real problem of a probiotic except for plasmid encoded antibiotic resistance like in E.faecium. It is important to emphasise the great value of supplementation with probiotics during antibiotic treatment in the prevention of Clostridia difficile diarrhoea and other complications associated with antibiotic treatment as discussed later in the text.

Clinical Aspects

Experiences from the clinic

As I have been working with many different patients during the last 10 years, there are a great number of stories to be told.

In general Probion given to people with disturbances from the gastrointestinal tract react very positively. What we often call a 'stress stomach' responds quite well after being administered Probion. Loose stools become normalised and constipated individuals suddenly experience a normalised defecation pattern i.e. 1-3 times daily. It is important to consider that initially, when beginning with probiotics, symptoms of unbalanced flora will be pronounced. This implies a slow and soft approach in most cases. Otherwise the individual could interpret these aggravations incorrectly. The more of an adjustment that you need, the more possible it is that these initiation symptoms will arise. These symptoms could be of any kind. They are related to the symptoms that are related to the dysbiosis itself, see all case reports beneath.

How to use Probion.

The Probion products are specially designed to adjust the microflora individually in different stages. Depending on every person's background it is advisable to balance the flora in certain levels. A recommended regime would be to initiate a probiotic therapy starting with a lower dosage. If the response is mild without any more pronounced side effects, it is possible to increase the dosage.

The decision how to approach this matter must be taken by the practitioner. Often it is more practical to start directly with Probion bifido in a low dosage. Patients with a condition and a history emphasising a more qualified intestinal dysbiosis need to start from a low level and should therefore be careful.

There is no difference between children and adults in general, though normally children do not have as severe dysbiotic conditions as can be the case in adults, so they do not need as much probiotics as grown up people.

However there are many individual variations and differences.

Most people will tolerate, to start with, 1 Tablet of Probion taken twice daily together with food. Increase the dosage to 2 tablets twice daily after one week. Some individuals would benefit from a dosage of 3-4 tablets twice daily. Another way to optimise could be to combine Probion and Probion bifido 2 tablets twice daily of each. If you are not sure how to start and if you are very sensitive, take 1 tablet in your mouth for a minute or two and then spit it out! As a rule begin slowly and test yourself towards the best dose.

Certain conditions when probiotics are of importance

Neurogenic diseases

Spinal muscular atrophy also called SMA. This is a genetic dependant disease amongst small children. Already in the first year of life, these children will be affected by an increasing atrophy of their nerve cells in the spinal cord. Their muscular capacity is markedly reduced. The disease is somewhat similar to the more well known Amyotrophic lateral sclerosis also called ALS. I was once contacted by a father, who told me that after about 7-10 days of taking Probion his child converted and started to stand up and walk. This was something that he had not been able to do for months. Taking the Probion away led to his earlier condition after a week. The procedure was repeated with the same manifestation! There certainly is a link between the microflora in the intestine and the immune system and the nervous system. What really happens is still to be explored. Clinical studies at the university hospital in Gothenburg are set up, but remain to be conducted due to lack of financial support. Meanwhile these children's nervous systems will continuously be affected without an optimal therapy.

Gastritis and ventricle ulcer, dyspepsia

These people respond quite quickly and they are therefore very grateful to treatment.

Constipation or colon irritable

Together with an adequate adjustment of the diet, these people need to start slowly with probiotics to achieve their objectives. Good results.

Migraine; conversion of tyrosine to tyrosamine

If related to diet there is an excellent effect.

Atopics i.e. eczema, hay fever, urticaria, asthma

Allergies are very complex immunological dysbalances. Probiotic approach will often give positive results. A friend taking all drugs there are for his asthmatic problems, also having some dyspeptic stress condition, converted in just one week after taking Probion! Now his need for medical drugs is close to nil. A change in diet is often needed.

Food intolerance e.g. glucose intolerance, lactose intolerance

If acquired by the use of antibiotics or other dysbiotic functions, these conditions often regress and vanish after a correct probiotic administration. Probiotic bacteria improve lactose digestion and increase enzyme activity in the intestine, which is an important step in preventing food allergies. Studies and practice have shown good results in these cases.

Chronic inflammatory disease or autoimmune diseases such as rheumatism, SLE, fibromyalgia, colitis ulcerosa, mb.Crohn etc.
As being related to a dysfunction in the immune system, adjusting the balance in the intestinal flora will give a good support in the recovery from these diseases.

Infections in the genito-urinary system
People with recidives or chronic infections are related to a dysbiosis. When taking the Probion there are many reports of reduced frequency or a total regress.

Mycosis i.e. Candida albicans
As being the top of the dysbiotic pyramid, this condition is corrected together with an adequate diet.

Exposition to radiation, cortisone, antibiotics, contraceptives
These ecological stress factors must be supported with probiotics, if to reduce the side-effects of these therapies.

Conditions with impaired immune defence i.e. malignant disease i.e. leucemias
These conditions need the support of probiotics.

Insufficiency of vitamins or minerals
All therapies with a nutritional impact must be supported by effective probiotics to increase the uptake of nutrients supplemented.

Stress
Maybe this is the most common condition. The need to adjust behaviour would naturally be supported by probiotics.

Skin diseases e.g. acne, herpes
The dysfunction of the endocrine system is often related to the intestinal flora. Herpetic infections are more complicated due to the intracellular nervous manifestation. Though these may respond as the outbreak of herpetic blisters is influenced of the general condition of the immune system.

Hormonal dysfunction i.e. bleedings, menstruation dysfunction, infertility and osteoporosis
As the hormonal balances in the body are influenced by the intestinal flora through the entero-hepatic linkage, problems of these natures would be adjusted by probiotic administration.

Metabolic syndrome and diabetes

There is a relation to the intestinal flora and to what you eat. Food with hyperglycaemic characteristics will influence both the flora and the conditions themselves. There are some reports indicating that some strains in the flora are able to produce insulin analogues. These may interfere with the normal insulin performance. It could even be a factor responsible to the development of insulin resistance!

Probiotics also reduce blood cholesterol.

Chronic fatigue syndrome

Antibodies against the intracellular mitochondria's are found to be of intestinal origin! These are thought to be responsible for this condition.

Diarrhoea

Products of microbial metabolism of dietary foodstuffs may also cause alterations of the mucosa. Such bacterial end products may be responsible for the diarrhoea and the colic which often accompany small bowel contamination.

The use of antibiotics is known to result in massive disturbances of the intestinal flora composition, often with long lasting negative effects including overgrowth by E.coli or other potential pathogens with resultant septicaemia and endotoxaemia. Diarrhoea thus is a common manifestation with patients receiving antibiotic therapy.

Everyday stress situations can also cause alterations in the quantity and composition of lactic-acid producing flora in the gastrointestinal tract. Diarrhoea frequently accompanies periods of nervous tension. This neurogenic diarrhoea is caused by excessive stimulation of the parasympathetic nervous system that greatly excites both motility and secretion of mucus into the colon.

Supplementation of probiotic bacteria have shown to decrease diarrhoea during antibiotic treatment (41) and improve the health of children with persistent diarrhoea (8).

Dysbiosis in man under extreme conditions was investigated (21). It was shown that yoghurt and other types of lactobacilli containing products could be used with success in order to minimise the disturbances caused in cosmonauts by the stress situations in long-term and short-term flights in space.

Neumeister (29) investigated the variations of normal bacterial flora in the small intestine during and after irradiation therapy in 500 patients with cancer. In order to eliminate some of the disturbances, 162 patients were administered orally a mixture of flora culture isolated from healthy human intestine and consisting of non-pathogenic E.coli, L.acidophilus and B.bifidus and pancreatic enzymes. The bacterial treatment was started at the same time as the X-ray treatment and continued during the whole treatment. Using X-ray therapy and supplementation with the lactobacilli preparation, the frequency of diarrhoea and other side effects decreased from 61 to 12% and in cobalt therapy from 79 to 21% which values are highly significant.

In gastro-enteritis where it can be an infection at any point of the gastrointestinal tract, in infectious diarrhoea, the infection is extensive in the large intestine. At any point of infection in the intestine, the mucosa becomes extensively irritated, and therefore its rate of excretion is enhanced. The motility of the intestinal wall is increased multifold, large quantities of fluids are made available for washing the infectious agent toward the anus with strong peristaltic waves. This is an important mechanism for ridding the intestinal tract of the debilitating infection. Lactobacilli can reverse this state, calm down the irritation of the mucosa and thus minimise the disturbance and diarrhoea.

In ulcerative colitis where also extensive areas of the intestinal wall of the large intestine is irritated and ulcerative, the motility is often increased as much as 10-fold, and the patient has repeated diarrhoeal bowel movements. During this state there is an impaired absorption of nutrients and a massive loss of fluids and electrolytes and thus a vicious circle for the patient.

Both during everyday stress and during extreme stress situations as well as infections the additional yoghurt intake with large amounts of viable lactobacilli may prove as beneficial in preventing and curing gastrointestinal disturbances (40).

Some final words

A quite new field in science is called psycho-neuro-immunology, which is the study of the interaction between psychological factors, the nervous system and the immune system. Since the intestinal microflora has such a strong influence on the immune system and also interacts with the hormonal system it could be said that there is a psycho-neuro-immuno-endocrino- intesto-microbiological linkage. In other words, all systems in the body are connected and a 'holistic thinking' is necessary in medicine, and recently proven thymic gland autonomic nervous system innervation and the potential effects thereof need to be taken into consideration.

Part 4 : Epilogue

4.1. Probiotics and Anti-Homotoxic Therapy.

Many suggestions have been made in this book, in respect of possible therapeutic uses of Probiotics i.e. suppression of diarrhoea, anti-tumour activity, stimulation of immunity etc. However, variant results on studies and trials are evident, and various factors may account for the differences in results, not the least being bio-individualistic/host specific.

Other factors to be considered are:

a) Type and strain of organisms in the probiotic.

b) Method of production, which may in turn affect ability of product to adhere to gut epithelium.

c) Amount and frequency of dosing, which may in turn affect 'fall off' after therapy ceases.

d) Viability of preparation in terms of numbers of viable organisms, and hence extent of quality control, and probably extent of effect of gastric acid destruction.

e) Original condition of gut microflora prior to probiotic administration and also the available matrix (NSP) prebiotic availability, nutrient availability to the flora (there is an argument in favour of Chlorella (cracked cell wall) supplementation alongside probiotics).

Research is continuing apace, and trials are also continuing: particular areas are:

1) Product, strains, viability, therapeutic protocols.

2) Determining how to maximise immuno-stimulatory effects and epithelial adherence factors.

3) Value of adjunct therapies and types of diet which enhance function.

4) Role of disrupters - not only antibiotics but endocrine disrupters such as organophosphates, herbicides, pesticides etc. from food and water, possibly additives (? Fluorine, chlorine etc.).

A few sources of these are listed below:

a) Steroids, NSAID's, alcohol.

b) Irritant foods, food intolerance's.

c) Toxins from altered gut bacteria and acquired bacteria.

d) Emotional stress from whatever source which tends to affect gut pH, and thus negatively influencing the flora.

e) Yeast's (Candida) and other parasites (e.g. Giardia).

Basically, and generally speaking in respect of the gut flora, most of the above can be considered as toxic effects. Thus, a link is established to a System of medicine called Homotoxicology, and the Anti-Homotoxic Therapy associated, utilising homoeopathically produced medicaments (combinations).

In June 1994 a seminar was conducted to seek a definition of Probiotics, and a team of international experts collaborated to develop the following definition:

"A probiotic agent is a microbial preparation containing live and/or killed microbes, including any constituent parts or metabolic products thereof. Probiotic agents may be employed as food additives, preventative substances or therapeutic substances."

Such provides a somewhat wider sphere and spectrum of therapeutic activity than hitherto indicated in this book. The mechanism of action, not only occurs directly with effects on the gut flora but also, as research continues with indirect effects on the mucosal immune system, the general immune system, the hormonal system, the nervous system and the metabolism.

Many controlled clinical tests have confirmed indications for microbiological therapy in wide spheres where immuno-modulation is considered desirable i.e. acute and chronic infections and autoimmune states, where the mucosal immune system of gut, lungs, urinary areas are involved. The preparation of Mucosa compositum (Heel), an example of Anti-Homotoxic Therapy, is an activator of these bodily defence mechanisms.

Alongside, though a major topic and study in it's own right, is the treatment of the toxin overload, known as detoxification therapy, utilising also homoeopathically prepared Anti-Homotoxic preparations according to a well established system 'Detox-Kit®' (Heel). Thus probiotic action is enhanced, as equally it should be by holistic integrative medicine approaches of lifestyle 'engineering' in terms of stress management and dietary/nutrient rebalance and ensuring the presence of total optimum nutrition to provide the precursors or exact nutrients for the body to possess ALL the necessary biological molecules for optimum immune system competence.

A brief on Homotoxicology According to Reckeweg is shown below:

Hans-Heinrich Reckeweg (1905 - 1985), the founder of the homeopathic pharmaceutical manufacturer "Biologische Heilmittel Heel GmbH" in Baden-Baden, Germany, developed a therapeutic method, in full knowledge of and including the homeopathic pharmacology with the so-called Homotoxicology, the theory of the homotoxins (homo = the human being, toxon = the poison), which attempts to reactivate the self-healing powers with the help of homoeopathically produced medicaments (combinations).

In his theory of Homotoxicology, Reckeweg defined every disease as a defence fight of the organism against exogenic toxins or against endogenic toxins which are created in the body by e.g. the metabolism. According to Reckeweg, disease is therefore always a dynamic occurrence and not a static one. In addition Reckeweg coined the term of the so-called vicariation; with this term he meant that a disease moves in phases through the homotoxicological Six-Phase Table which he developed.

In the Six-Phase Table he differentiates between humoral and cellular phases. The humoral phases are phases 1 to 3, the so-called excretion, inflammation, and deposition phases. They are separated from phases 4 to 6, the cellular phases, the impregnation, degeneration, and dedifferentiation phases, by the so-called "Biological Division".

If a disease is in one of the first three humoral phases, a healing "ad integrum" is almost always given, because all of the biological mechanisms of the body are fully functional. The toxins in the body are neutralised with the support of homeopathic medicaments, the so-called Anti-Homotoxic Preparations, and are flushed out of the body via the biological excretion channels of the body such as faeces, urine, sweat, spit, sputum, or also via abscesses and cysts. If, however, the biological mechanisms are no longer fully functional because of a too great toxin load, and the residual toxins remain therefore for longer periods of time in the tissues, these homotoxins can penetrate the cells and continue their destructive work there.

If a healing or at least a significant improvement of a disease of the cellular phase is to be achieved, the physician must direct his efforts to quasi shift the disease into a biologically safe disease from the first three humoral phases (proxy disease). Reckeweg calls this process a regressive vicariation effect.

If this is successful, the sick patient has the best chances for recovery. It is important, however, that the physician recognises this 'bio -logic' correctly and does not want to re-suppress the proxy disease with strong antidotes.

A vicariation phenomenon which often occurs exists among the skin disease, e.g. eczema and asthma. According to Reckeweg, asthma is a respiratory disease, especially of the bronchial tract, which is already in the impregnation phase. If this asthma is now excreted through a corresponding homeopathic treatment, it often vicariates into the form of an eczema.

If this eczema is then biologically cured with homeopathic medication, the asthmatic patient can recover fully. If the therapist is not aware of these connections and attempts to expel the eczema with an aggressive, suppressive- cortisone therapy, he usually shifts the more harmless skin disease back into the much more dangerous asthma. The patient then no longer has an eczema, but he has instead his asthma back!

Furthermore, the renowned Heringsche rule is hidden behind this vicariation phenomenon according to Reckeweg. It was named after Konstantin Hering, a student of Hahnemann's, who emigrated very early to the USA and became the founder of the American homeopathy. The so-called Heringsche rule says that every disease wanders from the outside to the inside and from the bottom to the top when it worsens and becomes a chronic disease thereby; chronic disease always heal from the inside to the outside and from the top to the bottom. As one can see, K. Hering too was aware of the connection that a skin disease arises during the healing of a chronic disease as the last phase of excretion of the chronic disease.

Unfortunately these connections are usually not known in traditional medicine and are not taken into consideration during therapy which results in the situation that we presently have a significantly higher proportion of chronically ill people than we had 60 years ago.

At the turn of the century the ratio of acute to chronic illnesses was approx. 80 to 20, these days it is the reverse. 80% of all illnesses are chronic and to more than 30% iatrogenically created damages which are generally caused by the highly effective but aggressive medicaments. The fact that this also has consequences for the ability to finance the health insurance systems is becoming more and more apparent in the Western industrial nations. There is not one country left in the EC which has not had to make considerable cutbacks in the social security system."

N.B. The author feels 'dedifferentiation phase' is better termed 'aberrant replication phase'.

Certain factors of modern day holistic biomedical science factors in the light of recent refined scientific methods and detailed, differentiated knowledge need to be considered for completeness.

I am grateful to Herzberger (2001) for these thoughts.

'The resulting fragmentation of medicine into specialities has led to advances in surgery and organ transplantation and in substitution therapy for metabolic disorders. But, the opposite development can be observed with the regard to the treatment of chronic conditions, such as vegetative regulatory disorders, cancer, rheumatic diseases and MS, in which multifactorial origins largely eliminate the possibility of treatment based on linear, causal reasoning. Thinking in terms of single causes provides at best a partial understanding of specialised processes. Thus, to find effective solutions to the problems of treating chronic illnesses, we have had to increase our understanding of dynamic interactions in biological systems, which - as information from the fields of cybernetics and open-system thermodynamics clearly demonstrates - are by no means linear but highly interconnected, and subject to a fluid state of biological balance, or 'steady state', because they constantly exchange energy and matter with their surroundings (Bertalanffy).

It is interesting that probiotics have proven themselves most effective in these chronic conditions and autoimmune states as equally in post antibiotic and cortisone, contraceptive pill states as innate immune system enhancers.

4.2 - Biological Parameters/ Epilogue

Research is proceeding apace today in so many spheres, in particular the spheres of immunology and molecular pathology, all of which reflect or present-day knowledge of intestinal micro-ecology and probiotic therapy, or create the need for further research into mucosal matters and the intestinal flora. Indeed, one of the problems of writing this book has been the constant input of ongoing research and the decision making as to what to include and what to leave to a 2nd edition. Also, so much is now known about intestinal microflora, another problem has been how to adequately present the ever-growing 'mountain of resource material' within the confines of page and pages space, yet produce a comprehensive, readable and practitioner useful volume.

It is hoped that my readers will excuse omissions, inaccuracies and lack of emphasis according to individual interests and likings, and seek to supplement their knowledge in such areas from specialist resource materials.

Undoubtedly, probiotics will expand in scope within medical and biological parameters in the future. Potentially exciting areas include vaccine development in humans and animals, perhaps also in respect of certain cancers. Certainly, probiotics (in the form of present-day strains or the development of new more specific or potent strains) have formed a niche of therapeutic modality, have become an integral functional food in the management of health in general, and have a role in alleviating the toxic, polluted, stress dominated world that surrounds the populace today. Let them become part of your practice.

So little done, so much to do....

References/Further Reading/Sources

Part I

1/ Natural Alternatives to Antibiotics. Leon Chaitow. Thorsons. 2001. ISBN 0-00-712247-0

2/ British Journal of Nutrition, Volume 80, No. 4, Oct. 1998, Including Supplement No. 2.

3/ Topics in Gastro Enterology, No. 7, Truelove/Willoughby, Blackwell Scientific Publications, 1979 - mainly out of date now.

4/ Micro-Ecology and Therapy, Vol. 10 - 1980, Institute for Micro-ecology, D6348, Herborn - Dill, Germany.

5/ Old Herborn University Seminar Monographs, Institute for Micro-ecology:
a)No. 1. Microbial Ecology of the Human Digestive Tract.
b)No. 8. Probiotics : Prospects of use in opportunistic infections.
c)No. 10. New Antimicrobial Strategies.
d)No. 11. Immunomodulation of the Gastrointestinal mucosa.

6/ Probiotics 2, Applications. Edited by Roy Fuller, Chapman and Hall, 1997, ISBN 0-412-73610-1

7/ Probiotics 3, Edited by R. Fuller, G. Perdigon, Immunomodulation by Gut Microflora and Probiotics, 2000, Kluwer Academic Publishers, ISBN 0-7923-6244-6

Part II

Dysbiosis - the (missing) link between health and disease - Lennart Cedgard M.D.

Ecology

?? Gastrointestinal microflora in mammalian nutrition. Ann. Rev. Nutr. 6:155-178, 1986. Savage D.C.

?? The composition of the faecal microflora in breast fed and bottle fed infants from birth to eight weeks. Actc Pediatr. Scand. 74:45-51, 1985. Lundeqvist B. et al.

?? Interactions among micro-organisms of the indigenous intestinal flora and their influence on the host. Rev. Infect. Dis. 6 suppl. 1. 573-9, 1984.

Nutrition

?? Contribution of Streptococcus thermophilus to growth-stimulating effect of yoghurt on rats. Dairy Sci. 63: 444-9, 1983. Wong et al.

?? The effect of yoghurt acidity on calcium bioavailability. 71st annual meeting March 29-April 2 exp. Biology, Washington D.C. 45(3) p.888, 1987. Kaup S.M. et al.

?? Yoghurt produces persistent increases in intestinal lactase activity. Clin. Res. 31(4) 764 A, 1983. Kolars J.C. et al.

?? Utilisation du calicium et du phosphore et mineralisation osseuse chez le porc consomment du yaourt. Sciences des aliments 6, p.15-30, 1986. Pointillart A.

?? Growth response of weaning rats to heated, aged, fractionated and chemically treated yoghurts. Dairy Sci. 63: 1065-72, 1980. Hargrove & Alford.

?? Lactose malabsorption from yoghurt, pasteurised yoghurt, sweet acidophilus milk and cultured milk in lactase deficient individuals. AM. CLJN NUTR 40(6), 1219-23, 1984. Savaiano et al.

Immunology

?? Intestinal microflora: the role of yoghurt in the equilibrium of the gut ecosystem. Int. J. Immunotherapy suppl. 2, 9-18, 1986. Bianchi-Salvadori B.

?? Possible treatment of Aids patients with live lactobacteria. Medical Hypotheses 26, 85-88, 1988. Tihole F.

?? The immunoregulation of the intestinal flora bifidobacteria and lactobacilli modulate the production of gamma-IFN induced by pathogenic bacteria. Int. J. Immunother. 3(2) 151-8, 1987. De Simone C.

?? Enhancement of immune response of murine Peyer's patches by a diet supplemented with yoghurt. Immunopharmacology and Immunotoxicology 9(1) 87-100, 1987. De Simone C.

?? Enhancement of immune response in mice fed with Streptococcus thermophilus and Lactobacillus acidophilus. J. Dairy Sci. 70:919-26, 1987. Perdigon G. et al.

?? Immunological responses to monassociated Bifidobacterium longum and their relation to prevention of bacterial invasion. Immunology 56(1) 43-50, 1985. Yamazaki S. et al.

?? Immunopotentiation of the mucosa of the small intestine of weaning piglets by peptidoglycan. Nippon Juigako Zasshi 49(2) 235-43, 1987. Sasaki T. et al.

?? Microflora yoghurt and the immune system JNT Immunother. 2(3) 9-18, 1986. De Simone C.

?? Mechanism of human complement activation by immunostimulators from bacterial cell walls. Bioorg. Khimiia 9(8) 1047-55, 1983. Kozlov L. V. et al.

?? The adjuvant effect of yoghurt on production of gamma interferon by con-A-stimulated human peripheral blood lymphocytes. NUTR REP INT 33(3) 419-34, 1986. De Simone C. et al.

?? Effects compares dùn regime enrichi en yoghourt vivant ou thermise sur le systeme immunitaire de la souris. Reprod. Nutr. Develop. 20(4A) 929-38, 1980. Conge et al.

?? Lactobacilli administered orally induce release of enzymes from peritoneal macrophages in mice. Milchwissenschaft 41(6) 344-8, 1986. Perdigon et al.

?? Effect of oral administration of lyzosome or digested bacterial cell walls on immunostimulation in Guinea pigs. Infect. Immun. 31(2) 580-3, 1981. Namba et al.

?? Microecology of the gastrointestinal tract and the immunological status under food allergy. Die Nahrung 28, 6/7, 689-93, 1984. Kuvaeva et al.

?? Immunopotentiating activity of orally-administered lactic bacteria, beneficial effect in infantile diarrhoea. Medicina (B. Aires) 46(6), 751-4, 1986. Perdigon et al.

?? Effects of Blastolysin and the glycopeptide muramyldipeptide N-Acetylglucosaminyl-muramyl dipeptide and carbohydrate fragments of peptidoglycans on human complement. Bioog. Khim. 11(11) 1510-18, 1985. Kozlov et al.

?? Immunochemical investigation of Blastolysine. Antibiot. Med. Biotekhnol. 30(4) 177-81, 1985. Bershadskaya et al.

Gastrointestinal system

?? Use of milk fermented with active bifidobacteria in the pregnant women. Med. Chir. Dig. Suppl. 3, no 16, 8-10. 1987. Ebissawa et al.

?? Effect of milk fermented with Bifidobacterium longum AB lab on digestive disorders and alterations of intestinal flora under antibiotic treatment. Med. Chir. Dig. Suppl. 3, no 16, 6-7, 1987. Colombel J. F. et al.

?? Clinical effects of bifidobacterium preparations on paediatric intractable diarrhoea. Keijo J. Med. 36(3), 298-314, 1987. Hotta M. et al.

?? Yoghurt with Bifidobacterium longum reduces erythromycin-induced gastrointestinal effects. Lancet vol. 2, 4/7 43, 1987.

Cancer

?? Antimutagenic properties of lactic acid cultured milk on chemical and faecal mutagens. J. Dairy Sci. 69(9), 2237-42, 1986. Hosono A. et al.

?? The metabolism of the intestinal microflora and its relationship to dietary fat, colon and breast cancer. Prog. Clin. Biol. Res. 655-85/222, 1986. Goldin B. R.

?? The effect of dietary fat and yoghurt on colonic bacterial enzymes (Beta-glucosidase and Beta-glucuronidase) associated with colon cancer. Food Microbiology 4;77-81, 1987. Cole C.B. & Fuller R.

?? Effects of feeding fermented milk on the incidence of chemically induced colon tumours in rats. Nutr. Cancer vol. 5 n:o 3-4 159, 1983. Shackleford L.A.

?? Lactobacillus overgrowth diet as an aid in controlling Escherichia coli septicaemia and endotoxaemia in cancer patients: a case report. J.American Geriatrics Soc. Vol. 18, n:o 5, 410-, 1970. Ellis S. et al.

Part 3.1.2

Correspondence to: Mark A. Brudnak, PhD, ND
Vice President, Technology
MAK Wood, Inc., 1235 Dakota Dr., Units E-F
Grafton, Wisconsin 53024-9429 USA
E-mail: makwood@earthlink.net

Part 3.2

1. Adams, M., and P. Marteau. 1995. **On the safety of lactic acid bacteria from food**. Int. J. Food Microbiol. 27:263-4.
2. Adlerberth, I., B. Carlsson, P. De Man, F. Jalil, A. R. Khan, P. Larsson, L. Mellander, C. Svanborg, A. E. Wold, and L. A. Hanson. 1991. **Intestinal colonisation with Enterobacteriaceae in Pakistani and Swedish hospital delivered infants**. Acta Paediatr Scand. 80:602-610
3. Adlerberth, I., B. Carlsson, L. Mellander, L. A. Hanson, F. Jalil, C. Svanborg. P. Larsson, and A. E. Wold. 1998. **High turn over rate of Escherichia coli strains in the intestinal flora of infants in Pakistan.** Epidemiol. Infect. In press:
4. Aguirre, M., and M. D. Collins, 1993. **Lactic acid bacteria and human clinical infection**. J Appl Bacteriol. 75:95-107.
5. Arunachalam, K., H. Gill, and R. K. Chandra. 2000. **Enhancement of natural immune function by dietary consumption of Bifidobacterium lactis (HN019).** Eur J Clin Nutr. 54:263-7.
6. Balmer, S. E., and B. A. Wharton. 1989. **Diet and faecal flora in the new-born: breast milk and infant formula.** Arch. Dis. Cild. 64:1672-1677.
7. Bennet, R., M. Eriksson, N. Tafari, and C.-E. Nord. 1991. **Intestinal bacteria of new-born Ethiopian infants in relation to antibiotic treatment and colonisation with potentially pathogenic Gram-negative bacteria.** Scand. J. Infect. Dis. 23:63-69.
8. Boudraa, G., M. Touhami, P. Pochart, R. Soltana, J. Y. Mary, and J. F. Desjeux. 1990. **Effect of feeding yoghurt versus milk in children with persistent diarrhoea**. J Pediatr Gastroenterol Nutr. 11:509-12.
9. Chaiken, B. 1994. **Yoghurt and autoimmune liver disease**. Am. J. Gastroenterol. Nutr. 89:1916-7.
10. Craig, S., and J. Cebra. 1971. **Peyer's patches: An enriched source of precursors for IgA-producing immunocytes in the rabbit.** J. Exp. Med. 134:188-200.

11. Dugas, B., a. Mercenier, I. Lenoir-Wijnkoop, C. Arnaud, N. Dugas, and E. Postaire. 1999. **Immunity and probiotics.** Trends of Immunology today. 20:387-390.
12. Elson, C., and W. Eadling. 1984. **Cholera toxin feeding did not induce oral tolerance in mice and abrogated oral tolerance to an unrelated protein antigen.** J. Immunol. 133:2892-2897.
13. Gallemore, G. H., R. T. Mohon, and D. A. Ferguson. 1995. **Lactobacillus fermentum endocarditis involving a native mitral valve**. J Tenn Med Assoc. 88:306-8.
14. Gasser, F. 1994. **Safety of lactic acid bacteria and their occurrence in human clinical infection.** Bull. Inst. Pasteur. 92:45-67.
15. Gorbach, S. 2000. **Probiotics and gastrointestinal health**. Am. J. Gastroenterol. 95:2-4.
16. Guy-Grand, D., C. Griscelli, and P. Vassalli. 1978. **The mouse gut T lymphocyte, a novel type of T cell. Nature, origin, and traffic in mice in normal and graft-versus-host conditions**. J Exp Med. 148:1661-77.
17. Helgeland, L., J. T. Vaage, B. Rolstad, T. Midtvedt, and P. Brandtzaeg. 1996. **Microbial colonisation influences composition and T-cell receptor V beta repertoire of intraepithelial lymphocytes in rat intestine.** Immunology. 89:494-501.
18. Kaila, M., E. Isoluri, E. Soppi, E. Virtanen, S. Laine, and H. Arvilommi. 1992. **Enhancement of the circulating antibody secreting cell response in human diarrhoea by a human Lactobacillus strain.** Pediatr Res. 32:141-4.
19. Kaizu, H., M. Sasaki, H. Nakajima, and Y. Suzuki. 1993. **Effect of anti oxidative lactic acid bacteria on rats fed a diet deficient in vitamin E.** J Dairy Sci. 76:2493-9.
20. Kim, J. H., and M. Ohsawa. 1995. **Oral tolerance to ovalbumine in mice as a model for detecting modulators of the immunologic tolerance to specific antigen.** Biol. Pharm. Bull. 18:854-858.
21. Lizko, N. 1987. **Stress and intestinal microflora**. Nahrung. 31:443-7
22. Majamaa, H., and E. Isolauri. 1997. **Probiotics: a novel approach in the management of food allergy**. J. Allergy Clin. Immunol. 99:179-85.
23. Majamaa, H., A. Miettinen, S. Laine, and E. Isolauri. 1996. **Intestinal inflammation in children with atopic eczema: faecal esinophil cationic protein and tumour necrosis factor-alpha as non-invasive indicators of food allergy.** Clin Exp Allergy. 26:181-7.

24. Marteau, P., M. Gerhardt, A. Myara, E. Bouvier, F. Trivian, and J. Rambaud. 1995. **Metabolism of bile salts by alimentary bacteria during transit in human small bowel.** Microbiol. Ecol. Health Dis. 8:151-7.
25. Matsuzaki, T., R. Yamazaki, S. Hashimoto, and T. Yokokura. 1998. **The effect of oral feeding of Lactobacillus casei strain Shirota on immunoglobulin E production in mice**. J Dairy Sci. 81:48-53.
26. Moore, W. E. C., and L. H. Moore. 1995. **Intestinal flora of populations that have a high risk of colon cancer**. Appl. Environ. Microbiol. 61:3202-3207.
27. Moreau, M., S. Hudault, and C. Bridonneau. 1990. **Systemic antibody response to ovalbumin in gnotobiotic C3H/HeJ mice with Bifidobacterium bifidum or Escherichia coli.** Microecol. Ther. 20:309-12.
28. Moreau, M.C., and G. Corthier. 1988. **Effect of gastrointestinal microflora on induction and maintenance of oral tolerance to ovalbumin in C3H/HeJ mice.** Infect. Immun. 56:2766-2768.
29. Neumeister, K. 1969. **Experimental therapy of intestinal radiation reactions in patients undergoing abdominal irradiation**. Radiobiol Radiother. 10:843-5.
30. Ouwehand, A. C., E. Isolauri, P. V. Kirjavainen, S. Tolkko, and S. J. Salminen. 2000. **The mucus binding of Bifidobacterium lactis Bb12 is enhanced in the presence of Lactobacillus GG and Lact.delbrueckii subsp.bulgaricus.** Lett Appl Microbiol. 30:10-3.
31. Parmely, M. J., and L. S. Manning. 1983. **Cellular determinants of mammary cell-mediated immunity in the rat: kinetics of lymphocyte subset accumulation in the rat mammary gland during pregnancy and lactation.** Ann N Y Acad Sci. 409:517-33.
32. Perdigon, G., S. Alvarez, M Nader de Marias, M. Roux, and A. Pesce de Ruiz Holgado. 1990. **The oral administration of lactic acid bacteria increases the mucosal immunity in response to enteropathogens**. J. Food Protect. 53:404-410.
33. Perdigon, G., M. E. De Macias, S. Alvarez, G. Oliver, and A. De Ruiz Holgado. 1986. **Effect on perorally administered lactobacilli on macrophage activation in mice**. Infect. Immun. 53:404-410.
34. Perdigon, ., M. E. De macias, S. Alvarez, G. Oliver, and A. De Ruiz Holgado. 1988. **Systemic augmentation of the immune response in mice by feeding fermented milks with Lactobacillus casei and Lactobacillus acidophilus.** Immunology. 63:17-23.

35. Roberfroid, M. 1996. **Functional effects of food components and the gastrointestinal system: chicory fructooligosaccharides**. Nutr. Rev. Nov 54:38-42.
36. Rotimi, V. O., S. A. Olowe and I. Ahmed. 1985. **The development of bacterial flora in premature neonates.** J. Hyg. Camb. 94:309-318.
37. Saxelin, M., N. Chuang, and B. Chassy. 1996. **Lactobacilli and bacteremia in Southern Finland, 1989-1992.** Clin. Infect. Dis. 22:564-6.
38. Saxelin, M., H. Rautelin, S. Salminen, and P. Makela. 1996. **Safety of commercial products with viable Lactobacillus strains**. Infect. Dis. Clin. Pract. 5:331-5.
39. Schroff, K., K. Meslin, and J. Cebra. 1995. **Commensal enteric bacteria engender a self-limiting humoral mucosal immune response while permanently colonising the gut**. Infect. Immun. 63:3904-3913.
40. Schultz, M., and R. Sarotr. 2000. **Probiotics and inflammatory bowel diseases.** Am. J Gastroenterol. 95:19-21.
41. Siitonen, S., H. Vapaatalo, S. Salminen, A. Gordin, M. Saxelin, R Wikberg, and A. Kirkkola. 1990. **Effect of Lactobacillus GG yoghurt in prevention of antibiotic associated diarrhoea.** Ann. Med. Feb; 22:57-9.
42. Sudo, N., S. Sawamura, K. Tanaka, Y. Aiba, C. Kubo, and Y. Koga. 1997. **The requirement of intestinal bacterial flora for the development of an IgE production system fully susceptible to oral tolerance induction**. J. Immunol. 159:1739-1745.
43. Van der Waaij, D., J, de Vries, and J. Lekkerkerk van der ees. 1972. **Colonisation resistance of mice during systemic antibiotic treatment**. J. Hyg. 70:605-609.
44. Yasui, H., N. Nagaoka, A. Mike, K. Hayakawa, and M. Ohwaki. 1992. **Detection of Bifidobacterium strains that induce large quantities of IgA**. Microbiol. Ecol. Health Dis. 5:155-62.

Part IV

1) Reckeweg, H.-H.: Materia Medica Homoeopathica Antihomotoxica, Vol. I, A Selective Pharmacology. Aurelia Publishers Ltd., Baden-Baden, Germany, 1996.

2) Reckeweg, H.-H.: Materia Medica Homoeopathica Antihomotoxica, Voll. II, Index of Symptoms and Modalities. Aurelia Publishers Ltd. Baden-Baden, Germany, 1991.

3) Bianchi, Ivo: The Principles of Homotoxicology. Aurelia Publishers Ltd., Baden-Baden, Germany, 1989.

4) Bianchi, Ivo: Homoeopathic Homotoxicological Repertory. Aurelia Publishers Ltd., Baden-Baden, Germany, 1995.

5) Journal of Biomedical Therapy (four issues a year), Official publication of SOHNA.

6) Further journals are available in different languages.

7) The Fundamentals of Homotoxicology. Gabriele Herzberger. 2001. Aurelia-Vertag.

For more literature about Homotoxicology, please contact:

The International Society of Homotoxicology (GB)
PO Box 217,
Ashford,
Kent, TN23 6ZU